MEETING

CARING FOR PERSONS LIVING WITH DEMENTIA AND THEIR CARE PARTNERS AND CAREGIVERS

A WAY FORWARD

Eric B. Larson and Clare Stroud, *Editors*

Committee on Care Interventions for
Individuals with Dementia and Their Caregivers

Board on Health Sciences Policy

Board on Health Care Services

Health and Medicine Division

A Consensus Study Report of

The National Academies of
SCIENCES · ENGINEERING · MEDICINE

THE NATIONAL ACADEMIES PRESS
Washington, DC
www.nap.edu

THE NATIONAL ACADEMIES PRESS 500 Fifth Street, NW Washington, DC 20001

This activity was supported by a contract between the National Academy of Sciences and the National Institute on Aging. This project was funded in whole or in part with federal funds from the National Institute on Aging, National Institutes of Health, U.S. Department of Health and Human Services, under Contract No. HHSN263201800029I. Any opinions, findings, conclusions, or recommendations expressed in this publication do not necessarily reflect the views of any organization or agency that provided support for the project.

International Standard Book Number-13: 978-0-309-15429-1
International Standard Book Number-10: 0-309-15429-4
Digital Object Identifier: https://doi.org/10.17226/26026
Library of Congress Control Number: 2021932470

Additional copies of this publication are available from the National Academies Press, 500 Fifth Street, NW, Keck 360, Washington, DC 20001; (800) 624-6242 or (202) 334-3313; http://www.nap.edu.

Printed in the United States of America

Cover credit: Original art reproduced with permission from Lenny Larson, who is living with dementia in Seattle, Washington.

Suggested citation: National Academies of Sciences, Engineering, and Medicine. 2021. *Meeting the challenge of caring for persons living with dementia and their care partners and caregivers: A way forward*. Washington, DC: The National Academies Press. https://doi.org/10.17226/26026.

The National Academies of

SCIENCES • ENGINEERING • MEDICINE

The **National Academy of Sciences** was established in 1863 by an Act of Congress, signed by President Lincoln, as a private, nongovernmental institution to advise the nation on issues related to science and technology. Members are elected by their peers for outstanding contributions to research. Dr. Marcia McNutt is president.

The **National Academy of Engineering** was established in 1964 under the charter of the National Academy of Sciences to bring the practices of engineering to advising the nation. Members are elected by their peers for extraordinary contributions to engineering. Dr. John L. Anderson is president.

The **National Academy of Medicine** (formerly the Institute of Medicine) was established in 1970 under the charter of the National Academy of Sciences to advise the nation on medical and health issues. Members are elected by their peers for distinguished contributions to medicine and health. Dr. Victor J. Dzau is president.

The three Academies work together as the **National Academies of Sciences, Engineering, and Medicine** to provide independent, objective analysis and advice to the nation and conduct other activities to solve complex problems and inform public policy decisions. The National Academies also encourage education and research, recognize outstanding contributions to knowledge, and increase public understanding in matters of science, engineering, and medicine.

Learn more about the National Academies of Sciences, Engineering, and Medicine at **www.nationalacademies.org.**

COMMITTEE ON CARE INTERVENTIONS FOR INDIVIDUALS WITH DEMENTIA AND THEIR CAREGIVERS

ERIC B. LARSON (*Chair*), Senior Investigator, Kaiser Permanente Washington Health Research Institute

MARILYN ALBERT, Professor of Neurology and Director, Division of Cognitive Neuroscience, Johns Hopkins University School of Medicine

MARÍA P. ARANDA, Associate Professor, Suzanne Dworak-Peck School of Social Work; Executive Director, Edward R. Roybal Institute on Aging, University of Southern California

CHRISTOPHER M. CALLAHAN, Chief Research and Development Officer, Eskenazi Health; Professor of Medicine, Indiana University School of Medicine

EILEEN M. CRIMMINS, AARP Professor of Gerontology and University Professor, Leonard Davis School of Gerontology, University of Southern California

PEGGYE DILWORTH-ANDERSON, Professor of Health Policy and Management, Gillings School of Global Public Health, University of North Carolina at Chapel Hill

XINQI DONG, Henry Rutgers Distinguished Professor of Population Health Science; Director, Institute for Health, Health Care Policy and Aging Research, Rutgers University

MIGUEL HERNÁN, Kolokotrones Professor of Biostatistics and Epidemiology, Harvard T.H. Chan School of Public Health

RONALD HICKMAN, JR., Associate Professor and Assistant Dean for Nursing Research, Frances Payne Bolton School of Nursing, Case Western Reserve University

HELEN HOVDESVEN, Co-Chair, Patient Family Advisory Council, Johns Hopkins Memory and Alzheimer's Treatment Center

REBECCA A. HUBBARD, Professor of Biostatistics, Department of Biostatistics, Epidemiology, & Informatics, University of Pennsylvania Perelman School of Medicine

JASON KARLAWISH, Professor of Medicine, Medical Ethics and Health Policy, and Neurology, University of Pennsylvania Perelman School of Medicine

ROBYN I. STONE, Senior Vice President for Research, LeadingAge

JENNIFER L. WOLFF, Eugene and Mildred Lipitz Professor; Director, Roger C. Lipitz Center for Integrated Health Care, Johns Hopkins Bloomberg School of Public Health

Advisors to the Committee

EVELYN FAVORS, care partner/caregiver, Washington, DC
CYNTHIA HULING HUMMEL, living with dementia, Elmira, New York
MARIE MARTINEZ ISRAELITE, care partner/caregiver, Chevy Chase, Maryland
RONALD LOUIE, care partner/caregiver, Seattle, Washington
KAREN LOVE, Dementia Action Alliance
JANET MICHEL, care partner/caregiver, Havre de Grace, Maryland
JOHN RICHARD PAGAN, living with dementia, Woodbridge, Virginia
BRIAN VAN BUREN, living with dementia, Charlotte, North Carolina

Study Staff

CLARE STROUD, Study Director
AUTUMN DOWNEY, Senior Program Officer
SHEENA POSEY NORRIS, Program Officer
ANDREW MARCH, Research Associate
PHOENIX WILSON, Senior Program Assistant (*until October 2020*)
KIMBERLY SUTTON, Senior Program Assistant (*from October 2020*)
BARDIA MASSOUDKHAN, Senior Finance Business Partner (*until September 2020*)
CHRISTIE BELL, Finance Business Partner (*from October 2020*)
ANDREW M. POPE, Senior Director, Board on Health Sciences Policy
SHARYL NASS, Senior Director, Board on Health Care Services

Consultants

RONA BRIERE, Senior Editor, Briere Associates, Inc.
THERESA WIZEMANN, Science Writer, Wizemann Scientific Communications, LLC

REVIEWERS

This Consensus Study Report was reviewed in draft form by individuals chosen for their diverse perspectives and technical expertise. The purpose of this independent review is to provide candid and critical comments that will assist the National Academies of Sciences, Engineering, and Medicine in making each published report as sound as possible and to ensure that it meets the institutional standards for quality, objectivity, evidence, and responsiveness to the study charge. The review comments and draft manuscript remain confidential to protect the integrity of the deliberative process.

We thank the following individuals for their review of this report:

BRUCE (NED) CALONGE, The Colorado Trust
ROBERT ESPINOZA, Paraprofessionals Healthcare Institute
DAVID GIFFORD, American Health Care Association
ANDREA GILMORE-BYKOVSKYI, University of Wisconsin School of Nursing
KATHY GREENLEE, Greenlee Global LLC
FRANCINE GRODSTEIN, Harvard Medical School and Brigham and Women's Hospital
LISA P. GWYTHER, Duke University
IAN KREMER, LEAD Coalition
TABASSUM MAJID, Intergrace Institute and University of Maryland, Baltimore County
KATIE MASLOW, Gerontological Society of America

SUSAN L. MITCHELL, Harvard Medical School and Hebrew Senior Life Institute for Aging Research in Boston
DAVID B. REUBEN, University of California, Los Angeles
NEELA PATEL, Glenn Biggs Institute for Alzheimer's & Neurodegenerative Diseases
PAUL B. SHEKELLE, University of California, Los Angeles, School of Medicine

Although the reviewers listed above provided many constructive comments and suggestions, they were not asked to endorse the conclusions or recommendations of this report, nor did they see the final draft before its release. The review of this report was overseen by **ENRIQUETA BOND,** Burroughs Wellcome Fund and QE Philanthropic Advisors, LLC, and **DAN G. BLAZER,** Duke University Medical Center. They were responsible for making certain that an independent examination of this report was carried out in accordance with the standards of the National Academies and that all review comments were carefully considered. Responsibility for the final content rests entirely with the authoring committee and the National Academies.

CONTENTS

PROLOGUE[1]

Cynthia Huling Hummel was diagnosed with amnestic mild cognitive impairment due to Alzheimer's disease in 2011. Her mother and uncle both died from Alzheimer's, and her grandmother had dementia. "The diagnosis changed my life," she said. She gave up her ministry because "I couldn't remember my parishioners or the experiences that we had shared together." She expressed frustration that it took 8 years and many visits to doctors to ultimately arrive at her diagnosis, after which she was sent off without any useful guidance.

Huling Hummel found that few programs were designed for persons navigating their diagnosis alone, and many services were unavailable to her as an individual without a care partner. "To me, that's not only demeaning, it doesn't recognize the fact that we're all different with our abilities," she said. Charting her own path, Huling Hummel built her own "circles of support" and began to focus on social interaction, spiritual support, and engaging in the arts, as well as exercise, healthy eating, and proper sleep.

[1] The vignettes presented here are from six persons living with dementia, care partners, and caregivers who spoke with the committee during open sessions in April and May 2020. They provided written permission to include their stories, quotes, and names. Many of the persons quoted here also advised the committee during the report writing phase, alongside several other individuals acknowledged in the report's front matter. While their stories are not intended to be representative of all experiences and views of persons living with dementia, care partners, and caregivers, their messages illustrate themes that underlie the body of research on dementia care and motivate the future directions recommended in this report, including urgency, complexity, diversity, individuality and personhood, community, love, and the importance of living life and finding joy.

After traveling this "lonely road," Huling Hummel felt called to work toward reducing the stigma associated with dementia, and to help others navigate the available supports, care, and services and "continue a life of purpose and joy." She emphasized that many persons living with dementia find music, art, and dance programs to be valuable resources that enhance their quality of life, and she encouraged the committee to consider biosocial and spiritual interventions and resources in its review.

John Richard (JR) Pagan lives with Lewy body dementia and autonomic dysfunction. Diagnosed about 7 years ago, he can no longer work, and he relies on his parents as care partners. Pagan pointed out that because of his age, he is not eligible for Medicare or Social Security retirement benefits. He observed that many studies of interventions focus on older people and those with more advanced disease, and he highlighted the lack of research attention to the needs of younger persons living with dementia and their care partners.

Still, Pagan is moving forward with his life, and he emphasized that psychotherapy has been an essential element of his ability to deal with the diagnosis of a progressive, terminal illness. "My therapist helped me to realize I'm living. I'm living today. I'm living tomorrow. Get out there and live life." As a moderator of a Lewy body dementia support group, Pagan has observed that "those of us that are having counseling, we're more resilient, we're more positive about our future." He noted that many people cannot access therapy because of cost, inability to travel to appointments, or lack of telehealth capability, and that those who are not developing resilience often struggle with severe depression, high anxiety, and suicidality. "These are very real issues," he said. Although research and evidence may be lacking in certain areas, Pagan hoped the committee would consider that "we are the lived experience of what is working."

Brian Van Buren is the third generation in his family to have Alzheimer's, having lost his mother, aunt, and both grandmothers to the disease. His own journey began 5 years ago when he was diagnosed with early-onset Alzheimer's disease. He described the experience as, "my doctor gave me the diagnosis, sent me home, basically to die." Van Buren has since become an active advocate. He served on the Alzheimer's Association Early-Stage Advisory Group, is involved with his North Carolina chapter of the Alzheimer's Association, and is an advisory board member of the Dementia Action Alliance. His advocacy work helped him realize that "if you hit a bump in the road you have two choices. You can either die or you can do something about it." Besides his advocacy work, he enjoys cooking and is an avid video streaming service fan.

Van Buren was a caregiver for his mother until her death 2 years ago at age 90. At one point, he cared for both her and his aunt, which he described as a personal and financial strain. He noted that many people quit jobs to care for family members at home because the cost of care facilities is prohibitive, adding that this can be a particular struggle for many African American families as they are acculturated to care for family members at home. Another cultural norm within African American families, he said, is not sharing that a loved one has Alzheimer's because of the shame associated with the disease.

Van Buren currently lives alone and does not have a caregiver. Instead, he has built a network of partners to help him navigate living with dementia, including a psychologist, a neurologist, a life coach, priests, a speech therapist, and others. "I kind of resent being told that I needed a caregiver," he said, "because that doesn't allow me to participate in my journey."

Marie Martinez Israelite once again became the caregiver for her mother after the COVID-19 pandemic caused her to move her mother out of an assisted living community. Her mother displayed behavioral and cognitive symptoms of dementia for about a decade and was diagnosed with Alzheimer's 4 years ago. Martinez Israelite, like many in the "sandwich generation," is balancing caregiving with her own work and family responsibilities. She added that it is common in communities of color for a grandparent living with dementia to reside long-term with family and observed that cultural dimensions of caregiving are generally not addressed in studies. She struggles to provide stimulating activities and social interaction to replace the activities her mother benefited from in assisted living and said, "I would really welcome any research that explores the best interventions and supports for families like mine."

Martinez Israelite expressed disappointment at the lack of conclusive evidence across the literature on dementia care interventions. She shared that she has experienced an overall improvement in her quality of life, including reduced distress, depression, and anxiety, from participating in a peer-to-peer support group. There is such great demand for these groups that she waited months before one had an opening for her to join. "I think of this twice monthly group as a lifeline," Martinez Israelite said. She also emphasized that exercise has been "critical to my mental health and my ability to muster the energy and coping skills necessary to help my mom effectively. People living with dementia and their families ... need multidimensional supports and tools to help cope with the medical and psychological challenges that we all encounter on this journey," she said.

Geraldine Woolfolk's professional achievements include conducting classes in music and English as a Second Language (ESL) in diverse older adult settings as an adult education teacher. In 1985 she helped lead the development of the first adult day social care program in the Oakland/East Bay region, which aimed to deliver extensive services to people living with dementia and provide respite for their caregivers. In the early 1990s, Woolfolk began caring for her mother, who developed dementia following a paralyzing stroke. Then, in the late 1990s, she found herself also caring for her husband, who was diagnosed with early-stage Alzheimer's disease. Her husband went from helping her care for her mother, assisting in music classes, and being a treasured volunteer at the day programs she helped create to becoming a program client himself. In 2007, his growing multi-faceted needs ultimately led to her placing him in a 48-bed care facility that was designed to exclusively serve people with dementia. She was extremely involved in his care and gave strong support to the medical and administrative staff in that specialized setting. Her husband passed away in 2012.

Woolfolk's professional and personal experiences continue to drive her passion for advocacy and for developing solutions to "help growing numbers of people of all generations who have to deal with the reality of either living with this condition or of caring for someone who does." Even with her professional background and wide network, Woolfolk said she still found it challenging to get information about comprehensive services in the community. More than two decades after her personal journey began, she finds that people today are still facing many of the same frustrations in getting information and caring for someone with dementia. She stressed that research needs to be translated into the development of relevant and seamless systems for providing practical information that can be used to support individuals and families that feel as if they are "swimming in the middle of the ocean with ... no life rafts." The number of people living with dementia is steadily growing, she said. "We *have* to do this.... We have to find a way to help them!"

Janet Michel is the caregiver for her husband, Kevin, who was diagnosed 10 years ago with mild cognitive impairment and more recently with Alzheimer's disease. Michel highlighted the value of disease education to persons living with dementia and their caregivers. "I need a lot of help dealing with nitty gritty things like bathing, giving meds, keeping my husband safe," Michel said. After Kevin's diagnosis, the couple joined the Johns Hopkins Patient and Family Advisory Council, where they began to learn about his disease, network, and attend conferences, which she found particularly helpful. "The more you know, the better caregiver you can be," she said. Being social and keeping active are also important to the couple, and Michel said it is helpful to understand that "others are going through the same thing that you are, in different ways." They joined an Alzheimer's support group and attend such activities as memory cafés, outings, and caregiver meetings. They also enjoy activities at the senior center, including dance classes, and Michel emphasized the benefits of music therapy. Unfortunately, the COVID-19 pandemic has disrupted many of these activities. Having a primary care provider who is knowledgeable about Alzheimer's disease and resources and who listens to both the patient and the caregiver is especially important when dealing with dementia, Michel said. Another need is respite care for caregivers, which can include other family caregivers, in-house care, adult day centers, and facility-based care for longer respite periods.

Overall, Michel said that "caregivers need down-to-earth, simple strategies that are available either in their home or close to their home," and she highlighted the importance of these being free or reimbursable. "We need to connect with people who are empathetic to our situation and who will help to lighten our burden physically, financially, and emotionally," she said. She urged the committee to remember that "it doesn't have to be perfect, but it really has to be soon."

PREFACE

At a time when unprecedented numbers of people are enjoying more years of life, this report of the National Academies of Sciences, Engineering, and Medicine describing a way forward for meeting the challenges of persons living with dementia and their care partners and caregivers could not be more timely and welcome. A previous National Academies study addressed the evidence on interventions to prevent or slow cognitive decline and dementia. The committee that conducted the present study was charged with reporting on evidence regarding interventions aimed at improving care for persons living with dementia and their care partners and caregivers. Both of these reports emanated from a widely shared desire to avoid dreading living to old age rather than approaching a long life as a reward for a life well lived.

In the waning decades of the 20th century, when the research world "discovered" late-life Alzheimer's disease and the importance of research to understand and address it, this developing field also recognized the need for quality improvement in caring for persons living with dementia, as well as their care partners and caregivers. Early advances led to findings that essentially helped reduce harm caused by unfortunately common practices in the care of persons with late-stage dementia. Examples included use of mechanical restraining devices (as exemplified by so-called "Geri-chairs") and chemical restraints, such as harmful overuse of antipsychotics. Today, Geri-chairs are virtually outlawed, and a recent report of the Lancet Commission documents declining use of antipsychotics. Likewise, harmful practices designed to sustain life, such as the use of feeding tubes and some other forced-feeding techniques, have declined significantly. Yet, while these changes represent progress, they can best be viewed as harm reduction due to existing practices.

While acknowledging the continuing need to reduce harm, a centrally important issue is how to move forward to focus on doing good and improving well-being. This report—sponsored by the National Institute on Aging (NIA) and based on a systematic review on the effectiveness of dementia care programs conducted under the auspices of the Agency for Healthcare Research and Quality (AHRQ)—addresses this issue of how to go beyond controlling behavior and addressing administrative regulations to focus on personhood and improving the well-being of both persons who develop dementia and their care partners and caregivers.

From the outset of this study, the committee members emphasized the importance of recognizing the unique disability—cognitive impairment—that characterizes those living with dementia, and of providing care aimed not just at accommodating that disability but also supporting whole-person care. This type of care is almost always complex and evolving. It must be offered in a way that maintains personhood, is guided by a focus on well-being, and considers other health conditions often seen in persons living with dementia. To better incorporate these principles into this study, the committee solicited substantial input throughout the study from persons living with dementia, care partners and caregivers, and advocacy groups, and this input was important in determining the ultimate content of the report. Also foundational to our efforts and this report are the guiding principles and core components of care detailed in Chapter 2.

The AHRQ systematic review on which this report is largely based identified thousands of published reports, many of which were rejected because they did not meet the review criteria. From this stringent review, two programs stood out: collaborative care programs and the REACH (Resources for Enhancing Alzheimer's Caregiver Health) trials. Collaborative care programs coordinate and integrate into ongoing primary care community resources and behavioral and mental health care. These programs can be seen as recognizing the complexity of caring for (mostly older) persons with dementia and of the needs of those providing that care. They recognize further that care needs evolve, and that the care provided can become chaotic and, in some cases, not serve the well-being of those who receive it. The REACH trials address the importance of providing care partners and caregivers with the knowledge, skills, and access to resources they need to promote their own well-being as well as that of the persons living with dementia for whom they care.

The committee was disappointed that the AHRQ systematic review did not uncover a stronger, more convincing evidence base. However, we want to highlight the many positive changes detailed in this report, including the shift in focus from avoiding harm to promoting well-being; recognition of the importance of conducting good research studies with an emphasis on rigor and generalizability; the development of collaborations; and, notably, incorporation of the perspectives of those experiencing dementia and their care partners and caregivers.

The last chapter of this report emphasizes the many opportunities for research and the implementation of its results to chart a way forward toward continued improvement in care that promotes the well-being of persons living with dementia and their care partners and caregivers. These opportunities include a recent increase in funding for such programs as the NIA IMbedded Pragmatic Alzheimer's disease and related dementias Clinical Trials (IMPACT) Collaboratory for embedded pragmatic trials, as well as promising areas for future research and implementation of proven interventions. We also note that during the committee's work, the COVID-19 pandemic disrupted the lives of all, but disproportionately those experiencing dementia and their care partners and caregivers. Just as every crisis contains an opportunity, the remarkable speed at which public science operated to develop vaccines and treatments, fueled by rapid increased funding for research and development, demonstrates just how valuable scientific research can be in advancing personal and public health. Together with strong support for public science, the findings identified in this report outline a way forward that will enable better care, and especially care that promotes the overall well-being of persons living with dementia and their care partners and caregivers. These ideas can serve as the basis for creating learning communities within care settings and society at large that will promote the notion that aging to late life is a reward rather than something to be dreaded.

This report resulted from the skill, expertise, and wisdom of a group of hard-working committee members, an able and supportive National Academies staff, and the input of diverse and dedicated stakeholders who offered their time and perspectives to the committee throughout this study. Thanks are extended to all.

Eric B. Larson, *Chair*
Committee on Care Interventions for Individuals with Dementia and Their Caregivers

ACKNOWLEDGMENTS

The committee would like to acknowledge and thank the study sponsor—the National Institute on Aging, and particularly Marie A. Bernard, Elena Fazio, Richard Hodes, Melinda Kelley, and Lis Nielsen—for their leadership in the development of this project. The committee gratefully recognizes and thanks Mary Butler, Joseph Gaugler, and the many others at the Minnesota Evidence-based Practice Center who worked on the preparation of the extensive Agency for Healthcare Research and Quality (AHRQ) systematic review that formed the primary evidence base used by the committee. The committee also thanks Kim Wittenberg and colleagues at AHRQ for their role in overseeing the systematic review.

The committee wishes to express its particular gratitude to the persons living with dementia, care partners, and caregivers who graciously shared their experiences, powerful thoughts, and advice with the committee, including Mary Radnofsky, who spoke at the committee's first meeting, and individuals who spoke with and advised the committee during the second phase of its work: Evelyn Favors, Cynthia Huling Hummel, Ronald Louie, Karen Love, Marie Martinez Israelite, Janet Michel, John Richard Pagan, Brian Van Buren, and Geraldine Woolfolk.

The committee also wishes to thank the many other individuals who gave presentations and participated in discussions with the committee, including Patrick Courneya (HealthPartners), Lynn Feinberg (AARP), David Gifford (American Health Care Association), Laura Gitlin (Drexel University), J. Neil Henderson (University of Minnesota), Kathleen Kelly (Family Caregiving Alliance), Shari Ling (Centers for Medicare & Medicaid Services), Douglas Pace (Alzheimer's Association), Lewis Sandy

(UnitedHealth Group), Richard Schulz (University of Pittsburgh), Melissa Simon (Northwestern University), Linda Teri (University of Washington), and Jennifer Weuve (Boston University).

Finally, the committee would like to express its gratitude to the National Academies staff who worked on the study: Clare Stroud, Autumn Downey, Sheena Posey Norris, Andrew March, Phoenix Wilson, and Kimberly Sutton. The committee is also grateful for the contributions of Theresa Wizemann, science writer; Rona Briere, editor; and Anne Marie Houppert and Maya Thomas of the National Academies Research Center for their assistance with fact checking.

SUMMARY[1]

Throughout the United States and around the world, millions of people are living with dementia, with impacts on their health and quality of life, on their families, and on society. The signs and symptoms of dementia can be a significant source of fear and distress for persons living with dementia, and many desire support in leading meaningful and rewarding lives, maintaining independence and agency, enjoying activities of interest, maintaining social relationships with others, and being connected to familiar environments and communities. To live well with dementia, people need care, services, and supports that reflect their values and preferences, build on their strengths and abilities, promote well-being, and address needs that evolve as cognitive impairment deepens. First may come support for decision making and engagement in pleasurable activities; followed by more extensive support in basic activities of daily living, such as eating and bathing; and potentially then by complete supportive care.

Persons living with dementia co-manage their care with or rely on the support of a wide range of care partners[2] and caregivers, including

[1] This Summary does not include references. Citations for the discussion presented in this Summary appear in the subsequent report chapters.

[2] "Care partner" is a term that refers to someone—often a family member, friend, neighbor, or group of individuals—with whom a person living with mild cognitive impairment (MCI) or early-stage dementia has a reciprocal relationship in co-managing the demands of MCI/dementia in such ways as providing emotional support and participating in decision making. Care partners may or may not live with the person or be involved in the provision of hands-on assistance with daily activities as a caregiver. Some persons living with MCI or dementia prefer the term "care partner" as it acknowledges the reciprocal contributions of and the partnership between both individuals.

spouses, other family members and friends, and direct care workers in homes or residential care settings, with the intensity of co-management changing over time. Those who provide care often experience positive aspects of caregiving, including a deeper appreciation for life, satisfaction with living according to one's values and sense of duty, and strengthening of their relationship with the person living with dementia. At the same time, however, caregivers also face higher risks to their physical and mental health, family conflict, social isolation, and negative consequences for their finances and jobs. Together, persons living with dementia and their care partners and caregivers need supports and services to help them live in a rewarding way.

Significant progress has been made in dementia care, services, and supports since the 1970s, when late-life dementia was not widely recognized as the consequence of a disease; diagnosis and treatment received little attention in the health care system; and care for persons living with dementia was largely considered a private family matter or, as a last resort, provided by state welfare systems in asylums and "old age homes." This progress is reflected in a rapidly expanding body of research; the 2011 National Alzheimer's Project Act; and the establishment of National Research Summits on Care, Services, and Supports for Persons with Dementia and Their Caregivers. Unfortunately, while there are places where persons living with dementia are receiving high-quality care, services, and supports, many lack access and are struggling and unable to live as well as they might. One study found that 99 percent of persons living with dementia living in the community and 97 percent of caregivers had at least one unmet need; the average number of unmet needs was 7.7 and 4.6, respectively, for persons living with dementia and caregivers. Deep and persistent inequities also characterize the care, services, and supports available to persons from disadvantaged groups, especially racial and ethnic minorities.

To help address this long-standing and deeply urgent need to better support persons living with dementia and their care partners and caregivers, there is a corresponding urgent need for evidence to guide effective action. In this context, the National Institute on Aging (NIA) requested that the National Academies of Sciences, Engineering, and Medicine convene an ad hoc committee of experts to assist NIA and the broader Alzheimer's disease and Alzheimer's disease–related dementias (AD/ADRD) community in assessing the body of evidence on care interventions for persons living with dementia and caregivers, inform decision making about which interventions should be broadly disseminated and implemented, and guide future actions and research.

ASSESSING THE STATE OF THE EVIDENCE

The body of evidence on care interventions, services, and supports (referred to here collectively as interventions for the sake of brevity) for persons living with dementia and their care partners and caregivers is large and complex. These interventions can be implemented at multiple levels—from individuals and families, to the community, to policy, to society—and delivered in diverse settings. Persons living with dementia and their care partners and caregivers are as diverse as the overall population, representing different ages, genders, races, ethnicities, sexual orientations, gender identities, and disabilities. In addition to the changes in needs that result from the progression of cognitive impairment, dementia care interventions themselves are often complex—they involve multiple components addressing aspects of daily life, health, planning and decision making, and relationships, and they interact with each other and with the context and system in which they are implemented. Hundreds of care interventions have been tested in randomized controlled trials (RCTs). While some interventions have been tested in large RCTs and are beginning to be implemented more broadly in various communities, many more have been tested only in academic settings with smaller numbers of participants. Thus, it is challenging to assess the current state of the evidence and understand what is effective, for whom, and under what circumstances.

In accordance with the study charge, the committee's primary source of evidence was a systematic review of the available RCT evidence on care interventions for persons living with dementia and their care partners and caregivers commissioned and overseen by the Agency for Healthcare Research and Quality (AHRQ) and conducted by the Minnesota Evidence-based Practice Center. The committee also considered additional evidence and stakeholder input, including perspectives from persons living with dementia, care partners, and caregivers, as described later in this summary.

The AHRQ systematic review provides a thorough review of available RCT evidence on care interventions for persons living with dementia and their care partners and caregivers. The literature search conducted for the AHRQ review also included prospective studies with concurrent comparator arms and interrupted time series with at least three measures both pre- and postintervention, but no such studies met the review criteria, and therefore these studies did not contribute to the review analysis. The AHRQ review is the product of a systematic and extensive effort to survey the body of literature and summarize the state of the evidence; it used clear criteria for including and excluding studies; it sheds light on the question of whether any interventions are supported by such conclusive and consistent evidence as to be immediately recommended for broad use without qualification or further study; and it provides a helpful overview of the evidence landscape.

It is important to emphasize that the AHRQ systematic review was designed specifically to inform the question of which interventions, if any, are ready for broad dissemination and implementation, and the AHRQ systematic review authors made decisions through this lens that inform the interpretation of the review findings and conclusions. The AHRQ systematic review excluded studies judged to be in Stages 0–II of the National Institutes of Health Stage Model for Behavioral Intervention Development (small-sample or pilot studies) and those judged to have high risk of bias.[3] Stages 0–II describe early-stage research that has not yet included testing of interventions in real-world settings. Excluding studies that have small sample sizes or high risk of bias is standard in systematic reviews. However, the exclusion of the heterogeneous category of pilots is important to interpreting the systematic review findings. While many pilots are small and preliminary, the review also excluded some studies that are described by the study authors as pilots although they used relatively large sample sizes (i.e., hundreds of participants), and in some cases were conducted in the community with longer follow-up times. Had the review targeted specific interventions in more depth and included research-setting efficacy studies without applying the lens of readiness for dissemination and implementation, the analysis and conclusions might have looked different. Because these pilot studies were not analyzed in the systematic review, it is unknown what portion of them could potentially be informative for efficacy and what portion would be excluded because of sample size or quality concerns.

The committee concluded that the evidence needed to inform decisions about policy and the implementation of specific interventions broadly—including prioritization of the many interventions that could be helpful but require resources—is limited. The AHRQ systematic review and this committee's analysis highlight limitations of the existing research base that can be addressed, such as a lack of diversity among study participants, underpowered and limited-duration studies, heterogeneity of outcome measures that precludes aggregation of results, lack of reporting on contextual factors that may facilitate or impede the effectiveness of interventions, and research that is divorced from practical implementation needs. Over time,

[3] Of the 627 unique studies eligible for analysis, 409 were excluded because they had small sample sizes or were pilots, and an additional 218 were assessed as having high risk of bias. Recognizing the challenges of conducting research in this area, the AHRQ systematic review authors set the sample size criterion generously: studies were excluded only if they had fewer than 10 participants per arm. Similarly, the review authors characterize their approach to assessing risk of bias as "generous, relative to how risk of bias is assessed in more targeted systematic review topics." For example, studies were assessed as having high risk of bias due to attrition only if attrition was greater than 40 percent.

standards for research are becoming more rigorous, but this progress is not yet fully reflected in the overall body of literature assessed in the AHRQ systematic review.

The inherent complexity of this area of study—including the importance of assessing interventions that target communities, policy, and society in addition to those that target individuals and families directly—also presents challenges to the evaluation of interventions and limited the AHRQ systematic review with respect to drawing conclusions. Mixed results observed across RCTs may reflect heterogeneity among enrolled populations, settings, or other contextual factors. Reflecting the wide range of needs, values, preferences, and desires of persons living with dementia, many interventions in this domain appropriately begin from the premise of individualization. It is to be expected that the effectiveness of interventions will vary across different populations and settings. Furthermore, many factors beyond effectiveness that are critical for successful implementation, such as integration into workflow, may vary across settings, but these differences may be obscured as results are synthesized in a broad-scope systematic review. Thus, it is currently impossible to determine through a high-level systematic review whether an intervention is ineffective, whether it is effective but only for some people or in certain settings, or whether only some of its elements are effective.

Consistent with its charge, the committee relied heavily on the findings from the AHRQ systematic review. That review identified no interventions that met its criteria for high-strength or moderate evidence of benefit and just two types of interventions supported by low-strength evidence of benefit: (1) collaborative care models, which use multidisciplinary teams that integrate medical and psychosocial approaches to the care of persons living with dementia; and (2) a multicomponent intervention aimed at supporting family caregivers known as REACH (Resources for Enhancing Alzheimer's Caregiver Health) II, along with associated adaptations.

The findings of the AHRQ systematic review with regard to intervention effectiveness were used to identify the above two types of interventions as potentially ready for broad dissemination and implementation. In addition to effectiveness, however, many factors need to be considered in determining whether broad implementation of an intervention is appropriate. To inform the development of its recommendations on these two types of interventions, the committee applied the GRADE (Grading of Recommendations Assessment, Development and Evaluation) Evidence to Decision (EtD) framework to the interventions identified by the systematic review as being supported by low-strength evidence of benefit. Factors taken into account in this framework include the priority of the problem, how substantial the benefits and harms of the intervention are, the certainty of the evidence, the value of the outcomes to stakeholders, how the intervention compares with others, resource requirements, cost-effectiveness relative to comparable options, the impact on health equity, the acceptability of the intervention to stakeholders, and the feasibility of implementation. Information for the application of this framework was culled from studies of various adaptations and implementations of the two types of intervention. The AHRQ review authors rated some of these implementation studies as having high risk of bias and excluded others because they used methodologies that failed to meet the review's inclusion criteria, such as studies with a single pre–posttest. Nevertheless, these studies provide such information as feasibility, equity, and resources required, which is important for making decisions about implementation in the real world. The committee identified these additional studies by reference mining the studies that met the AHRQ review inclusion criteria, reviewing studies mentioned in the AHRQ review that did not meet the inclusion criteria, conducting PubMed and hand searches, and reviewing the Best Practice Caregiving database and Center for Medicare & Medicaid Innovation evaluations of dementia care interventions.

Taken together, these studies provide a rich source of evidence beyond the outcomes on which the AHRQ review was able to draw conclusions. Thus, without negating the AHRQ review's conclusions regarding the low strength of evidence or the uncertainties that prevented the review from reaching conclusions on many outcomes, the committee deemed that compiling the comprehensive set of available evidence on effectiveness could be informative for those considering implementing these two types of interventions in a range of settings.

Finally, to inform its conclusions about gaps in the current evidence base and opportunities for moving forward, the committee considered input and information beyond that included in the AHRQ systematic review. A systematic review is necessarily limited to existing literature, and therefore reflects past research priorities. In particular, the perspectives of persons living with dementia, care partners, and caregivers have historically not been central in guiding research. Recognizing the importance of changing this situation, the committee sought to identify opportunities to expand the evidence base for interventions deemed important by persons living with dementia, care partners, and caregivers. The committee also considered other expert and stakeholder input presented during a public workshop and such resources as the Best Practice Caregiving database, which aided in the identification of types of interventions already being implemented in real-world practice settings but for which the AHRQ systematic review found insufficient evidence of effectiveness.

MOVING TOWARD BETTER DEMENTIA CARE, SERVICES, AND SUPPORTS

The charge to this committee was to examine the available evidence on specific interventions for providing dementia care, services, and supports to inform policy, institutional/community decisions about broadly implementing interventions, and prioritization of the many interventions that could be helpful but require resources that are limited. Unfortunately, the evidence to inform this task is lacking. This does not mean, however, that fundamental principles or core components of dementia care, services, and supports are called into question. Rather, it points to the need for additional research to fill gaps in information about specific interventions. In the interim, organizations, agencies, communities, and individuals can use the guiding principles in Box S-1 and the core components of care in Box S-2 to guide their actions toward improving dementia care, services, and supports. Given the critical need for improvements in the current situation, access to care, services, and supports that followed these principles and included these components would represent a significant advance for persons living with dementia and their care partners and caregivers.

Furthermore, there are many activities, such as listening to music and dancing, that provide pleasure for many people living with or without dementia and likely have little potential harm apart from opportunity and financial costs. At an individual or family level, persons living with dementia and their care partners and caregivers may want to experiment with these types of activities, tailored to their personal interests and preferences, to see what works for them, knowing this may change as the condition progresses.

INTERVENTIONS READY FOR IMPLEMENTATION IN REAL-WORLD SETTINGS WITH MONITORING, EVALUATION, QUALITY IMPROVEMENT, AND INFORMATION SHARING

Together, the two types of interventions identified by the AHRQ systematic review as supported by low-strength evidence of benefit—collaborative care models and REACH II and associated adaptations—incorporate many, although not all, of the core components of care, services, and supports listed in Box S-2.

Collaborative Care Models

Collaborative care models use multidisciplinary teams to integrate medical and psychosocial approaches to the care of persons living with dementia. These programs—such as ACCESS, Dementia Care Management,

BOX S-1
Guiding Principles for Dementia Care, Services, and Supports

The following principles can guide ideal care, services, and supports for persons living with dementia and their care partners and caregivers. Unfortunately, their application is currently limited.

Person-centeredness: Recognition of persons living with dementia as individuals with their own goals, desires, interests, and abilities.

Promotion of well-being: The use of social, behavioral, and environmental interventions that holistically address the needs of persons living with dementia, care partners, and caregivers to enhance well-being.

Respect and dignity: Attention to each person's particular needs and values, which can be achieved by following models for identifying preferences and values, such as values elicitation, shared decision making, respect for dissent, or seeking either assent or informed consent.

Justice: Treating people with equal need equally so that, for example, all critically ill persons receive critical care, all expectant mothers receive prenatal care, and the dying receive palliative care. By extension, all persons living with dementia, care partners, and caregivers have equal access and can receive care, supports, and services according to their needs.

Racial, ethnic, sexual, cultural, and linguistic inclusivity: The availability of racially, ethnically, sexually, culturally, and linguistically appropriate services for all who may need them, especially underserved and underrepresented populations, such as racial and ethnic minorities and LGBTQ individuals.

Accessibility and affordability: Care, services, and supports for persons living with dementia, care partners, and caregivers that do not impose an unmanageable financial burden on individuals or their families and are available and accessible to all who may need them, including those living in rural communities.

Care Ecosystem, and the Indiana University/Purdue University Model—have multiple common components, including coordination of psychosocial interventions, medical management, and other services through a care manager; the development of care plans; case tracking; and collaboration with care providers. Aggregating results across collaborative care interventions to draw conclusions regarding particular outcomes, the AHRQ systematic review found sufficient evidence to support conclusions of low-strength evidence that collaborative care models are effective for three outcomes for persons living with dementia: (1) quality of life, (2) quality indicators,

BOX S-2
Core Components of Care, Services, and Supports for Persons Living with Dementia and Their Care Partners and Caregivers

Several existing frameworks describe core components of ideal dementia care, supports, and services that promote the well-being of persons living with dementia, care partners, and caregivers. The components listed below are ideally designed with the participation of the individuals involved, managed throughout the course of the condition, and adjusted according to the many changes experienced by persons living with dementia and their care partners and caregivers:

- Detection and diagnosis
- Assessment of symptoms to inform planning and deliver care, including financial and legal planning
- Information and education
- Medical management
- Support in activities of daily living
- Support for care partners and caregivers
- Communication and collaboration
- Coordination of medical care, long-term services and supports, and community-based services and supports
- A supportive and safe environment
- Advance care planning and end-of-life care

NOTE: Descriptions of these components and sources are provided in Chapter 2.

and (3) emergency room visits. In addition to the outcomes for which the AHRQ systematic review found low-strength evidence of benefit, both the systematic review and original study authors identified evidence of benefit for other outcomes in individual studies, including decreasing neuropsychiatric symptoms and nursing home placement for persons living with dementia, and reducing caregiver strain and depression. The evidence was not sufficient to warrant reaching conclusions on effectiveness for these outcomes, generally because of inconsistent findings across studies.

A Multicomponent Intervention for Family Caregivers: REACH II and Adaptations

REACH II is a multicomponent intervention that provides support for family care partners/caregivers through a combination of strategies that include problem solving, skills training, stress management, support groups, provision of information and education, and role playing. It has been adapted for different populations and for delivery in different settings across the United States and elsewhere, including Germany and Hong Kong.

The AHRQ systematic review found that there is low-strength evidence that REACH II and its adaptations reduce caregiver depression. Although the available evidence was insufficient to draw a conclusion, the systematic review also identified a reduction in caregiver strain. Additional studies of adaptations of REACH II that did not meet the AHRQ review inclusion criteria illustrate trends in benefits on a wide range of other outcomes, including challenging behaviors of persons living with dementia, caregiver frustration or bother, and physical symptoms of psychiatric conditions. Studies of adaptations of REACH II also found improvements in self-reported social support, self-reported caregiver health, caregiver reactions to challenging behaviors, positive aspects of caregiving, and safety of persons living with dementia. Although the AHRQ systematic review did not find sufficient evidence to support conclusions about these outcomes, the trends of benefit across many outcomes in these implementation and adaptation studies complement the AHRQ systematic review findings.

Recommendations

Collaborative care models and REACH II and its adaptations have demonstrated some effectiveness under clinical trial conditions. Both—but especially REACH II and its adaptations—are already being implemented in a variety of community settings with promising results. Of particular note, REACH II has been studied in and adapted for diverse populations to a greater extent than is usual in the field. The original trial studied the intervention in a study population that was one-third Black or African American, one-third white or Caucasian, and one-third Hispanic or Latino, although it did not include Asian participants. Later adaptation studies have also been conducted with racially and ethnically diverse study populations, with linguistic and cultural adaptations, and with low-income participants and communities. A moderate amount of evidence is available with respect to intervention acceptability, feasibility, and resource requirements. Collaborative care models and REACH II and its adaptations are ready for the next stage of field testing to support their widespread adoption in and adaptation to the variety of settings where people seek care, and to enhance understanding and information dissemination regarding key factors beyond effectiveness that are important for determining whether and how to implement such an intervention.

The state of the evidence base for these two intervention types as assessed by the AHRQ review complicates making recommendations for a path forward. The AHRQ finding of low-strength evidence of effectiveness suggests limited confidence in the effectiveness of these interventions and indicates that additional evidence is likely to change the estimate of effect. Nevertheless, the committee recommends a path forward based on the following argument. First, given the inherent challenges of studying this topic—including the complexity of dementia care interventions, the diversity of populations affected, and the importance of contextual effects—the fact that these two interventions produced low-strength evidence of effectiveness is important. Second, there is a notable trend in benefits across multiple outcomes beyond those for which the AHRQ review was able to draw a conclusion, and the consistency of evidence of benefit across sources of evidence is encouraging. Third, there is a moderate amount of evidence to inform implementation as assessed against the EtD criteria. Particularly important, these interventions have been studied in diverse populations, although additional evidence is needed to expand understanding of their use in all populations.

Taken together, these considerations led the committee to conclude that the evidence is sufficient to justify implementation of these two types of interventions in a broad spectrum of community settings, with evaluation conducted to continue expanding the evidence base to inform future implementation. The committee believes that this approach to expanding the evidence base is likely to bring greater gains and better inform real-world implementation relative to focusing on additional large RCTs aimed at generating moderate- or high-strength evidence in a future systematic review before any further dissemination can be supported.

RECOMMENDATION 1: *Implement and evaluate outcomes for collaborative care models in multiple and varied real-world settings under appropriate conditions for monitoring, quality improvement, and information sharing.*

To enhance the evidence base for decision making about the implementation of collaborative care models—which use multidisciplinary teams to integrate medical and psychosocial approaches to the care of persons living with dementia—agencies of the U.S. Department of Health and Human Services (HHS) should work with state Medicaid programs and health care systems to implement these interventions and evaluate their outcomes in multiple and varied real-world settings under appropriate conditions for monitoring, quality improvement, and information sharing. Along with adding to the current evidence for effectiveness, these efforts should include examining key factors that are important for determining whether and how to implement an intervention, such as identifying workforce and space needs, testing payment models and integration into workflow, and ensuring adaptations for different populations (e.g., racial/ethnic

groups) and settings (e.g., rural areas). Specifically, to advance these efforts:

- The Centers for Medicare & Medicaid Services should explore the value of collaborative care models offered as a benefit through Medicare Advantage programs and alternative payment models and for fee-for-service beneficiaries to build the infrastructure, train the workforce, and redesign the workflows that would facilitate the adoption, monitoring, and evaluation of these programs.
- State Medicaid programs serving persons living with dementia and dual-eligible beneficiaries should encourage participating health systems, systems that provide long-term services and supports, and managed care organizations to provide collaborative care for persons living with dementia. This care could be included in a dementia-focused quality metric.
- The National Institute on Aging, HHS's Office of the Assistant Secretary for Planning and Evaluation, the Agency for Healthcare Research and Quality, and the Administration for Community Living should support research and stakeholder engagement focused on collaborative care models to aid in scaling and sustaining the models; identifying monitoring and evaluation standards; developing monitoring and evaluation plans; and sharing information about key findings, lessons learned, and promising practices.
- Health care systems, including those in the U.S. Department of Veterans Affairs, should support infrastructure that would facilitate the collaboration of providers of primary care, mental health and other specialty care, and long-term services and supports within the health care system and with local home-based community services and supports agencies in implementing collaborative care models to improve the well-being of persons living with dementia and their care partners and caregivers.

RECOMMENDATION 2: *Implement and evaluate outcomes for REACH II and its adaptions in multiple and varied real-world settings under appropriate conditions for monitoring, quality improvement, and information sharing.*

To enhance the evidence base for decision making about the implementation of REACH II and its adaptations—a multicomponent intervention that provides support for family care partners and caregivers—agencies within the U.S. Department of Health and

Human Services (HHS) should work with state agencies, community organizations, and care systems to implement and evaluate outcomes of these interventions in multiple and varied real-world settings under appropriate conditions for monitoring, quality improvement, and information sharing. Along with adding to the current evidence for effectiveness, these efforts should include examining key factors that are important for determining whether and how to implement an intervention, such as identifying workforce and space needs, testing payment models and integration into workflow, and ensuring adaptations for different populations (e.g., racial/ethnic groups) and settings (e.g., rural areas). Specifically, to advance these efforts:

- The Centers for Disease Control and Prevention and the Administration for Community Living should incorporate REACH II and its adaptations into its efforts to support evidence-based dementia programs at state and local public health departments in concert with community organizations.
- The Centers for Medicare & Medicaid Services should explore the value of REACH II and its adaptations offered as a benefit through Medicare Advantage programs and alternative payment models and for fee-for-service beneficiaries to build the infrastructure, train the workforce, and redesign the workflows that would facilitate the adoption, monitoring, and evaluation of these programs.
- State Medicaid programs serving persons living with dementia and dual-eligible beneficiaries should encourage participating health systems, systems that provide long-term services and supports, and managed care organizations to provide REACH II and its adaptations for care partners and caregivers. This care could be included in a dementia-focused quality metric.
- The National Institute on Aging, HHS's Office of the Assistant Secretary for Planning and Evaluation, the Agency for Healthcare Research and Quality, and the Administration for Community Living should support research and stakeholder engagement focused on REACH II and its adaptations to aid in scaling and sustaining the model; identifying monitoring and evaluation standards; developing monitoring and evaluation plans; and sharing information about key findings, lessons learned, and promising practices.
- The U.S. Department of Veterans Affairs should participate in monitoring, quality improvement, and information-sharing

initiatives to enable other entities to learn from its implementation of this intervention.

- **Health care systems should support infrastructure that would facilitate the collaboration of providers of primary care, mental health and other specialty care, and long-term services and supports within the health care system and with local home-based community services and supports agencies in implementing REACH II and its adaptations to improve the well-being of persons living with dementia and their care partners and caregivers.**

It is important to stress that these recommendations should not be taken to imply that these are the only two types of interventions that should be pursued. As discussed next, additional research on a full range of interventions should be undertaken to continue to innovate and develop better ways of meeting the urgent needs of persons living with dementia and their care partners and caregivers.

THE STATE OF THE EVIDENCE FOR OTHER DEMENTIA CARE INTERVENTIONS: GAPS AND OPPORTUNITIES

Beyond the two types of interventions discussed above that met the AHRQ systematic review's criteria for low-strength evidence of benefit, the review found insufficient evidence to support conclusions about benefit for all other interventions. Importantly, a finding of insufficient evidence does not necessarily mean that an intervention is ineffective, but rather reflects high uncertainty given the limitations of the evidence base and of the approach used in the AHRQ systematic review to synthesize the existing evidence and assess its strength to support conclusions on readiness for broad dissemination and implementation. As described above, the limitations of the existing evidence base are due in part to the inherent complexity of this area of study, but some of these limitations can be addressed.

The evidence base for dementia care interventions appears biased toward those targeting the individual level. The gap in the evidence base for interventions targeting the community, policy, or societal level—such as organization, financing, and delivery processes—may result from the way researchers define interventions and the challenges of studying these latter kinds of interventions with rigor, which may necessitate expanded or alternative approaches to studying and assessing evidence.

In addition, there remain significant gaps in the evidence base for many individual-level interventions evaluated in the AHRQ systematic review, some of which have been identified by persons living with dementia, care partners, and caregivers as important to their health and well-being, such as respite care, social support, late-stage care, and training and support for direct care workers. There is a lack of evidence as well regarding the effectiveness of dementia care interventions in diverse populations, such as specific racial/ethnic groups; LGBTQ populations; people with significant comorbidities; people of low socioeconomic status; and those from low-resource areas, such as rural and tribal populations. Variation in the experiences and circumstances of persons living with dementia and their care partners and caregivers may also have implications for the perceived value of interventions, the fidelity of implementation, and intervention effectiveness that need to be better understood. Consequently, the applicability of the existing evidence base to the full range of persons living with dementia, care partners, and caregivers is not supported, even for those interventions showing promise in clinical trials.

Finally, the evidence for some intervention categories—such as exercise, music, psychosocial interventions, and cognitive interventions—is insufficient to support conclusions on their readiness for broad dissemination and implementation despite a signal of benefit. Signal of benefit was determined based on the observation of benefit for a given outcome in multiple independent RCTs evaluating the same (or a similar) intervention, even if the overall body of evidence was mixed for that outcome (i.e., one or more RCTs found no benefit for that outcome). As a result of heterogeneity in study populations, intervention implementation, and measured outcomes, little is known regarding which interventions are likely to be effective for persons living with dementia experiencing different stages of disease progression and their care partners and caregivers, and how they should be optimally implemented.

A BLUEPRINT FOR FUTURE RESEARCH

To strengthen the evidence base by addressing the limitations described above, the committee offers a blueprint for future research. This blueprint includes methodological improvements aimed at limitations frequently found in the current evidence base—such as underpowered and limited-duration studies, and heterogeneity of outcome measures that precludes aggregation across studies—as well as approaches that can supplement the quantitative measures in RCTs to advance understanding in the face of the complexity of dementia care interventions and the systems in which they operate. To ensure that research is representative, generalizable across populations, and person-centered, the committee stresses the importance of prioritizing inclusive research and incorporating the priorities of persons living with dementia, care partners, and caregivers throughout the study process. Finally, the committee emphasizes the need to expand the focus on community- and policy-level interventions and to conduct research aimed at assessing key factors in determining real-world effectiveness.

RECOMMENDATION 3: *Use strong, pragmatic, and informative methodologies.*
When requesting applications and identifying funding priorities for research on care interventions for persons living with dementia and their care partners and caregivers, the National Institute on Aging and other interested organizations should prioritize strong, pragmatic, and informative methodologies that take account of this complex domain, including studies that

- ensure a balanced portfolio of short- and longer-term studies with sufficient sample size;
- use a harmonized core of outcomes and a taxonomy of interventions to enable pooling of study findings;
- focus on outcomes of greatest priority to persons living with dementia and their care partners and caregivers, including intended and unintended benefits and harms, across the continuum of early- through late-stage dementia;
- include qualitative methods in studies that have quantitative outcomes;
- use observational study methods to complement randomized trials; and
- commit to comprehensive study reporting to enable improving and better understanding fidelity, studying context effects, and learning from negative results and unsuccessful methodological approaches.

RECOMMENDATION 4: *Prioritize inclusive research.*
When funding research on care interventions for persons living with dementia and their care partners and caregivers, the National Institutes of Health (NIH) and other interested organizations should prioritize research that promotes equity, diversity, and inclusion across the full range of populations and communities affected by dementia through studies that

- are conducted by broadly inclusive research teams;
- include racially, ethnically, culturally, linguistically, sexually, and socioeconomically diverse participants by requiring adherence to the NIH Revitalization Act of 1993, and assess disparities in access and outcomes; and
- use study designs that support inclusivity.

RECOMMENDATION 5: *Assess real-world effectiveness.* When funding research on care interventions for persons living with dementia, care partners, and caregivers, the National Institutes of Health, the Agency for Healthcare Research and Quality, the Centers for Medicare & Medicaid Services, the Administration for Community Living, and other interested organizations should support research capable of providing the evidence that will ultimately be needed to make inclusive decisions and implement interventions in the real world, including studies that, to the extent possible,

- **improve the assessment of individual-level interventions by leveraging complementary study methodologies;**
- **expand the focus on community/policy-level interventions using a broad set of research methodologies; and**
- **address key factors (e.g., space, human resources, work redesign, and adaptations) that need to be taken into account to assess the real-world effectiveness of these interventions.**

To address the long-standing and urgent need to better support persons living with dementia and their care partners and caregivers in living as well as possible, there continues to be an urgent need to build a more robust and useful evidence base. Studying dementia care interventions is challenging and complex, and the body of evidence is complicated to interpret. Two types of interventions are supported by sufficient evidence for implementation in real-world settings with evaluation to continue to expand the evidence base. These interventions are practical instantiations of many of the core components of care, supports, and services discussed above, which are needed to promote the well-being of persons living with dementia and their care partners and caregivers. Given current major deficits in the care, services, and supports that are available now, providing these interventions to those who could benefit would be a step forward. Yet, this is not a final answer. It is important that research continue to develop and evaluate other potentially promising interventions, many of which have demonstrated some signal of benefit. The committee's recommendations provide a path forward for building a more robust and useful evidence base by employing cutting-edge methods that are rigorous, most informative for this domain, inclusive, and equitable, and can yield information critical for real-world implementation. These exciting approaches can be implemented throughout this field, including by early-career researchers and others who want to harness new approaches to make a difference in addressing this critical societal need and better supporting persons living with dementia and their care partners and caregivers in living as well as possible.

1

INTRODUCTION

Throughout the United States and around the world, millions of people are living with dementia, with impacts on their own health and quality of life, on their families and other caregivers, and on society more broadly. The signs and symptoms of dementia can be a significant source of fear and distress for persons living with dementia, and many desire support in leading meaningful and rewarding lives, maintaining independence and agency, enjoying activities of interest, maintaining social relationships with others, and being connected to familiar environments and communities (Gitlin and Hodgson, 2018; Han et al., 2016). To live as well as possible, persons living with dementia need medical care, physical quality of life, social and emotional quality of life, and access to services and supports. The needs, values, preferences, and desires of different individuals vary and evolve over time. In its early stages, persons living with dementia may need support in such activities as planning, making decisions, attending medical appointments, and engaging in pleasurable community and social activities. As cognitive impairment progresses, persons living with dementia need more extensive care and support in such basic activities of daily living as eating and bathing and in oversight of medications and more complex medical care, as well as continued support in engaging in activities that bring pleasure. Finally, as with many progressive diseases, some persons living with dementia will enter a terminal phase in which complete supportive care is needed.

Because of the disease's effects on the ability to perform daily activities, persons living with dementia co-manage its demands with or rely on the support of a wide range of care partners and caregivers, including spouses, other family members, friends, and direct care workers in the home or in care settings, working individually or in combination. These care partners and caregivers may or may not reside with the person living with dementia, who may live alone, particularly during their condition's early stages. And as the needs of the person with dementia evolve over time, so, too, does the intensity of co-management.

Those who provide care often experience positive aspects of caregiving, including a deeper appreciation for life, satisfaction with living according to one's values and sense of duty, and strengthening of the relationship between the care partner or caregiver and the person living with dementia (NASEM, 2016; Roth et al., 2015). However, caregivers also face higher risks to their physical and mental health, family conflict, social isolation, and negative consequences for their finances and jobs. Neither unpaid nor paid caregivers—direct care workers such as home health aides or certified nursing assistants—receive adequate training and support for this challenging work (Burgdorf et al., 2019; NASEM, 2016). Alongside persons living with dementia, care partners and caregivers require their own services and supports to live well themselves.

Significant progress has been made in the care, services, and supports provided for persons living with dementia, care partners, and caregivers since the 1970s, when dementia was not widely recognized as the consequence of a disease; diagnosis and treatment received little attention in the health care system; and care for persons living with dementia was largely a private family matter or, as a last resort, provided by state welfare systems in asylums and "old age homes." The need for quality care and supports for persons living with dementia, as well as support for their care partners and caregivers, is now recognized as a fundamental societal issue, as highlighted in two of five primary goals in the National Plan to Address Alzheimer's Disease (ASPE, 2020).

Research on care interventions for persons living with dementia and for care partners and caregivers has expanded greatly in the past three decades, and some care-related programs are starting to be disseminated and implemented more broadly (Gitlin et al., 2015; Mitchell et al., 2020). Yet, while there are places where persons living with dementia and their care partners and caregivers are receiving and delivering high-quality care, many are still struggling, lack access to care interventions, and are unable to live as well as they might (NASEM, 2016). Furthermore, it is well known that, compared with non-Hispanic whites, racial and ethnic minorities, such as Blacks, Hispanics, and American Indians/Alaska Natives, have both a higher prevalence and incidence of Alzheimer's disease and other dementias (Dilworth-Anderson et al., 2008; Gilsanz et al., 2019; Mayeda et al., 2016; Steenland et al., 2016) and less access to care for these conditions, including diagnosis, treatment, and supports (Gianattasio et al., 2019;

Rivera-Hernandez et al., 2019). Furthermore, racial disparities persist in the care persons living with dementia receive. For example, while such harmful practices as the use of feeding tubes in individuals with advanced dementia has decreased in recent years, feeding tube use has remained significantly higher in Black compared with white individuals (Mitchell et al., 2016). Research suggests that Black caregivers may demonstrate greater resilience and may be less likely to experience emotional difficulty (Fabius et al., 2020), and that African American and Hispanic caregivers report more positive attitudes toward caregiving (Dilworth-Anderson et al., 2020). Nonetheless, caregivers in racial/ethnic minority groups, especially women, are also at greater risk of experiencing the financial challenges associated with caregiving (Kelley et al., 2015; Willert and Minnotte, 2019). Despite the progress made in recent decades, then, it is clear that this journey to improve care, services, and supports for persons living with dementia, care partners, and caregivers remains an urgent need.

The body of evidence on care interventions for persons living with dementia and their care partners and caregivers is large and complex. Hundreds of interventions have been tested in randomized controlled trials (RCTs) (Butler et al., 2020; Gitlin et al., 2015). These interventions are designed for persons across all stages of dementia, from early through severe; for different caregivers, including family members, friends, and direct care workers; and for implementation in many settings, including the home and home health care, social service agencies, and institutional settings. In addition, while some interventions have been tested in large RCTs and are beginning to be implemented more broadly in various communities, many more have been tested in academic settings with smaller numbers of participants.

STUDY CHARGE AND SCOPE

In this context, the National Institute on Aging (NIA) requested that the National Academies of Sciences, Engineering, and Medicine convene an ad hoc committee of experts to assist NIA and the broader Alzheimer's disease and Alzheimer's disease–related dementias (AD/ADRD) community in assessing the body of evidence on care interventions for persons living with dementia and caregivers,[1] inform decision making about which interven-

[1] The Statement of Task for this study does not specifically mention "care partners," a term that refers to individuals who collaborate with persons living with dementia, particularly during the early stages of the disease when they are able to co-manage their own care to a greater extent. Such individuals have previously been encompassed by the term "caregiver;" however, the committee opted to distinguish care partners from caregivers in recognition of their different roles and the reciprocal nature of the relationship between persons living with dementia and care partners.

tions should be broadly disseminated and implemented, and guide future actions and research. The committee's Statement of Task is presented in Box 1-1; Box 1-2 contains definitions for key terms used in this report; and biographical sketches of the committee members and staff are provided in Appendix C.

In accordance with its charge, the committee used as its primary source of evidence a systematic review of evidence on care interventions for persons living with dementia and their care partners and caregivers commissioned and overseen by the Agency for Healthcare Research and Quality (AHRQ) and conducted by the Minnesota Evidence-based Practice Center (EPC) (Butler et al., 2020). The committee also considered additional evidence and stakeholder input, including perspectives from persons living with dementia, care partners, and caregivers, as described in the section on methods below and further in Chapter 5.

BOX 1-1
Statement of Task

An ad hoc committee will assess the evidence on care-related interventions for people with dementia and their caregivers, and make recommendations to inform decision making about disseminating and implementing care interventions on a broad scale. The committee's work will be based on a systematic review commissioned by the Agency for Healthcare Research and Quality (AHRQ) and is taking place in two phases. In the first phase, which has been completed, the committee provided input into the design of the AHRQ systematic review in the form of a letter report that describes potential changes to and considerations for the preliminary systematic review key questions and scope.

In this second phase, after the AHRQ systematic review is released, the committee will reconvene to consider the evidence found. The committee's scope will be based on the final key questions and scope of the AHRQ systematic review, which will address care interventions relevant to Alzheimer's disease and Alzheimer's disease–related dementias (AD/ADRD, to include Lewy body dementia, frontotemporal dementia, and vascular cognitive impairment/dementia). The committee will hold an information-gathering workshop open to the public during the course of its work to seek input from stakeholders on the draft AHRQ report. Based predominantly on the AHRQ systematic review, as well as on this additional expert and public input, the committee will assess the quality of existing evidence and develop a detailed report that makes recommendations to inform the National Institute on Aging and the AD/ADRD community (including, but not limited to, persons living with dementia and their families, and their health care providers) regarding whether sufficient evidence exists for care/nonpharmacologic interventions that are ready for dissemination and implementation on a broad scale. The report will also identify gaps in relevant fields of research that the National Institutes of Health may wish to explore further.

The scope of this study and the AHRQ systematic review was broad. It encompassed interventions relevant to individuals with possible or probable AD/ADRD—including Lewy body dementia, frontotemporal dementia, and vascular cognitive impairment/dementia—at all stages of dementia. The scope also included care partners and caregivers who are related to the person living with dementia, such as spouses, family members, friends, and volunteers, as well as direct care workers, such as certified nursing assistants, home health aides, auxiliary workers, personal care aides, hospice aides, promotoras or promotores, and community health workers.

The scope encompassed a wide range of care interventions whose primary target is persons living with dementia, care partners and caregivers, or both together, such as memory evaluation, art therapy, social support, skills training, changes to the physical environment, care coordination, and many more (see Box 1-3 for a full list of examples). Recognizing the multidimensional nature of dementia care, services, and supports, the scope encompassed the wide range of outcomes that are relevant to the health and well-being of persons living with dementia and their care partners and caregivers, including outcomes related to quality of life and subjective well-being, personal and family spending and financial burden, health and functional status, palliative care/hospice, the social/community level, utilization and costs of health care services, quality of care and services, societal costs, and harms (see a full list in Appendix A and in Butler et al., 2020). The scope encompassed as well a full range of settings and services, including home health care, adult day care, acute care settings, social service agencies, nursing homes, assisted living, memory care units, hospice, rehabilitation centers/skilled nursing facilities, long-distance caregiving, and nonplace-based (virtual) settings.

Neither the study nor the systematic review examined pharmacological treatments for dementia, supplements, or natural products. And while it is important to recognize that many persons living with dementia, care partners, and caregivers have other chronic conditions for which they need care, this study did not consider evidence for nonpharmacological interventions that many persons living with dementia may use for other conditions, such as continuous positive airway pressure (CPAP) machines. The systematic review also excluded interventions to provide training toward professional licensing or continuing education for degreed health professionals. Finally, although outcomes related to utilization and costs of health care services were included when reported by the original study authors, a cost-effectiveness analysis was outside the scope of the AHRQ systematic review and this study.

BOX 1-2
Key Terminology Used in This Report

The appropriate terms to use in discussing dementia care are the subject of debate among the many stakeholders involved and are also shifting. Indeed, dementia-related terminology, nomenclature, and stigma was a major theme of the 2017 National Research Summit on Care, Services, and Supports for Persons with Dementia and Their Caregivers. Thus, it is challenging to select clear and consistent terms that will reflect the preferences and lived experiences of all or even a majority of the readers of this report. Acknowledging the differences in terms used and preferred by different stakeholder groups, the committee opted to use the terms defined below. The selection of these terms is not intended to be an endorsement of these particular terms or their definitions, but to explain how the terms are used in this report.

Person living with dementia: A person living with dementia is an individual living with Alzheimer's disease or Alzheimer's disease–related dementias (AD/ADRD). Dementia results from at least one of a variety of diseases, the most common being neurodegenerative diseases such as Alzheimer's disease, Lewy body dementia, frontotemporal dementia, and vascular cognitive impairment/dementia. Dementia describes disabling cognitive impairments, which progress over time. A person living with dementia needs assistance with performing one or more daily activities.

Person living with mild cognitive impairment (MCI): This term denotes an individual living with cognitive impairment that has reached a level relative to normal cognitive function that is identifiable by individuals, family members, or clinicians, but without significant functional impairment in the performance of daily activities (i.e., the individual may have mild functional impairments such that he or she is less efficient with functional tasks but can adapt to those impairments).

Care partner: A care partner is someone with whom a person living with MCI or dementia has a reciprocal relationship in co-managing the effects of dementia in such ways as providing emotional support and supporting decision making. Care partners are often family members, but may also be neighbors, friends, or fictive kin (individuals with a close relationship with but unrelated by birth, adoption, or marriage to persons living with dementia). Care partners may or may not be involved in the provision of hands-on assistance with daily activities as a caregiver. Some persons living with MCI or dementia prefer the term "care partner" as it emphasizes the strengths and abilities of each person and acknowledges the partnership between them.

Caregiver: Caregivers may be family members, neighbors, friends, fictive kin, or any other individual providing unpaid health- and function-related assistance to persons living with dementia. The term "caregiver" may be used more frequently in the care of a person living with dementia as the person experiences more disabilities.

Direct care workers: These paid caregivers provide hands-on long-term care and personal assistance to persons who are living with disabilities. They include nursing assistants and nursing aides, who generally work in nursing homes and other residential care settings; home health aides, who provide personal care and some health-related assistance to people who typically need postacute, short-term skilled nursing care in their homes or in community settings; personal care aides who deliver nonmedical services in private or group homes; and promotoras/promotores ("promoters of health" in Spanish-speaking communities) and community health workers.

Clinicians: The term encompasses physicians, psychologists, nurses, advanced practice providers, pharmacists, physical therapists, occupational therapists, social workers, and other skilled health care workers who are credentialed to care for individual patients. They are licensed by states.

Care interventions, services, and supports: This term denotes an array of paid and unpaid personal care, health care, and social services and supports generally provided over a sustained period of time. They are delivered by health care, social services, and other community organizations or care partners and caregivers with the intent of having a direct impact on either persons with dementia or their caregivers/care partners or both. They encompass supports, services, programs, accommodations, or practices that include behavioral, environmental, technological, and psychological methods or approaches, including long-term services and supports (LTSS) for personal care (e.g., bathing or dressing) and help with instrumental activities of daily living (such as medication management, paying bills, transportation, meal preparation, and health maintenance tasks). They can be provided in a variety of settings, such as nursing homes, residential care facilities, adult day centers, and individual homes, and contribute to a person's well-being, happiness, identity, privacy, capacity, autonomy, or authority.

Long-term services and supports (LTSS): LTSS encompass the broad range of paid and unpaid medical and personal care assistance that people may need to accommodate a short- or long-term disability. They may be provided in nursing and other residential care facilities or in a broad range of community settings, including individuals' homes or apartments.

Care system: In this report, the term refers to the systems that provide health care and long-term care services and supports, which encompass, respectively, medical care and the full range of long-term care and other social services and supports, such as respite care, adult day activity programs, and transportation. These services and supports include the expertise of clinicians, such as physicians, psychologists, nurses, therapists, and social workers, in settings that include the hospital, primary care office, clinic, and community.

Care team/network: The care team/network consists of persons living with dementia and their family members or friends (when desired by the person living with dementia), all professionals providing health care and long-term services and supports, and other social services professionals who interact with individuals in their care.

SOURCES: Butler et al., 2020; NASEM, 2016, 2017; Sferrazza, 2020.

BOX 1-3
Example Interventions Included in the AHRQ Systematic Review

- Memory evaluation
- Driving evaluation or encouraging driving cessation
- Meaningful activities
- Advance care planning
- Behavior management
- ADL support
- Home modifications
- Wandering and fall risk management
- Palliative care
- Caregiver support and support groups
- Sensory-based interventions
- Changing the physical environment/environmental modification across settings (e.g., in hospitals, in people's homes)
- Mindfulness training
- Interventions focused on the development of Dementia Friendly Training (e.g., training of police officers in local communities)
- Wandering and wayfinding
- Reminiscence therapy
- Prompts and multicomponent interventions
- Engagement interventions
- Exercise interventions
- Psychoeducational
- Art therapy
- Dance movement therapy
- Music therapy
- Cognitive behavior therapy
- Counseling/care management (including emotionally focused couples therapy)
- General support
- Respite
- Training of PLWD
- Psychosocial interventions/studies
- Caregiver support groups
- Therapeutic counseling
- Support interventions, including involving informal caregiver social network to support the primary caregiver
- Cognitive reframing (changing caregivers' maladaptive behaviors or beliefs)
- Web-based multimedia intervention
- Caregiver-therapist e-mail support
- Educational and peer-support website
- Bereavement support
- Improving acute care systems
- Skill training, including for CNAs, home health aides, and/or informal caregivers
- Training for CNAs, home health aides, and/or informal caregivers
- Improving care transitions
- Care coordination
- Multicomponent interventions

NOTE: ADL = activity of daily living; CNA = certified nursing assistant; PLWD = people living with dementia.
SOURCE: Excerpted from Butler et al., 2020, pp. A-1–A-2.

METHODS

The committee first met in November 2018 to provide input into the design of the AHRQ systematic review. This meeting included an open session in which NIA provided the committee's charge, leaders from the Minnesota EPC team presented the draft key questions and scope for the systematic review, and the committee invited dementia-related advocacy groups to offer their perspectives (Appendix B includes the agendas for all open sessions held for this study). The committee authored a brief letter report to outline its input for the review design (NASEM, 2018), after which the Minnesota EPC developed a draft review protocol, which was discussed with the committee during a public meeting in February 2019.

Over the next year, the Minnesota EPC conducted the systematic review, and a draft was publicly released in March 2020. The committee reconvened in April 2020 to discuss this draft. This meeting included a day-long workshop, held virtually because of the COVID-19 pandemic. The workshop included presentations by and discussions with representatives from the Minnesota EPC review team; advocacy organizations and associations representing persons living with dementia, care partners, and caregivers; care systems and payers; and academic science. In May 2020, the committee met with a group of persons living with dementia, care partners, and caregivers to hear their perspectives on the draft systematic review and gather their input for this report.

The committee continued to meet virtually over the spring, summer, and fall of 2020, and the final AHRQ systematic review was published in August 2020. The committee's September 2020 meeting included a brief open session with leaders from the Minnesota EPC and other interested parties to discuss the final version of the systematic review. In addition, a group of persons living with dementia, care partners, and caregivers—some of whom also had participated in the May 2020 open session—served as advisers to the committee during the drafting of this report (see the list of these advisers in the front of the report).

AHRQ Systematic Review Design

The AHRQ systematic review provides a thorough review of evidence from available RCTs on care interventions for persons living with dementia and their care partners and caregivers. The literature search conducted for this review also included prospective studies with concurrent comparator arms and interrupted time series with at least three measures both pre- and postintervention, but no such studies met the review criteria, and therefore these studies did not contribute significantly to the review analysis. Box 1-4 summarizes the methodology of the review, key questions addressed,

BOX 1-4
Description of the AHRQ Systematic Review

Review Methodology

Objective. To understand the evidence base for care interventions for people living with dementia (PLWD) and their caregivers, and to assess the potential for broad dissemination and implementation of that evidence.

Data sources. We searched Ovid Medline, Ovid Embase, Ovid PsycINFO, CINAHL, and the Cochrane Central Register of Controlled Trials (CENTRAL) to identify randomized controlled trials, nonrandomized controlled trials, and quasi-experimental designs published and indexed in bibliographic databases through March 2020.

Review methods. We searched for nondrug interventions targeting PLWD, their informal or formal caregivers, or health systems. Two investigators screened abstracts and full-text articles of identified references for eligibility. Eligible studies included randomized controlled trials and quasi-experimental observational studies enrolling people with Alzheimer's disease or related dementias or their informal or formal caregivers. We extracted basic study information from all eligible studies. We assessed risk of bias and summarized results for studies not judged to be National Institutes of Health (NIH) Stage Model 0 to II (pilot or small sample size studies) or to have high risk of bias. We grouped interventions into categories based on intervention target.

Key Questions

The Agency for Healthcare Research and Quality (AHRQ) systematic review developed 10 key questions to guide the research and organize the literature. These key questions are organized by four broad intervention categories and subsequently by the target of the intervention and population in which outcomes are being evaluated. The 10 key questions adhere to the following structure:

For **PLWD** _or_ family and/or paid **PLWD caregivers,** what are the benefits and harms for

- Care interventions aimed at treating the behavioral and psychological symptoms of dementia (BPSD) in PLWD?
- Care interventions aimed at improving quality of life, function, or non-BPSD symptoms in PLWD?
- Care interventions aimed at supporting the quality of life and health outcomes of the family and/or paid PLWD caregivers?
- Care delivery interventions?

Each key question also included the following supplemental questions: (1) what evidence is available on how outcomes differ by **PLWD** _or_ family and/or paid **PLWD caregiver** characteristics? and (2) which intervention characteristics or components are associated with effectiveness?

Summary of Inclusion Criteria

The AHRQ systematic review included studies that enrolled adults of any age with possible or diagnosed AD/ADRD. Studies could include individuals with mild cognitive impairment if they constituted less than 15 percent of the study population or if results for PLWD were reported separately. Studies were included if they reported on any of the outcomes addressed in the key questions above. The AHRQ review included randomized controlled trials and prospective studies with a concurrent comparator arm, and at least 10 participants in each arm at the time of study analysis. Interrupted time series with at least three measures both pre- and postintervention were also included. Studies that were published in English in either peer-reviewed journals or as grey literature with the full-text article available were included.

Grading the Strength of Evidence

The overall strength of evidence was evaluated based on five required domains: (1) study limitations (risk of bias); (2) consistency (similarity of effect direction and size); (3) directness (single, direct link between intervention and outcome); (4) precision (degree of certainty around an estimate); and (5) reporting bias. Based on these factors, we rated the overall strength of evidence for each outcome as:

- High: Very confident that estimate of effect lies close to true effect. Few or no deficiencies in body of evidence, findings are believed to be stable.
- Moderate: Moderately confident that estimate of effect lies close to true effect. Some deficiencies in body of evidence; findings likely to be stable, but some doubt.
- Low: Limited confidence that estimate of effect lies close to true effect; major or numerous deficiencies in body of evidence. Additional evidence necessary before concluding that findings are stable or that estimate of effect is close to true effect.
- Insufficient: No evidence, unable to estimate an effect, or no confidence in estimate of effect. Available evidence or lack of evidence precludes judgment.

Notably, an assessment of insufficient evidence does not mean that the intervention is ineffective. Rather, it means that due to the uncertainty of the evidence, we could not draw meaningful conclusions about its effectiveness at this time.

NOTE: Terminology and abbreviations used in this box are those of the AHRQ systematic review and do not necessarily correspond to the terminology used in this report.
SOURCE: Excerpted from Butler et al., 2020, pp. vii, 18–19. For the inclusion criteria, see also Appendix A.

inclusion criteria for studies, and strength-of-evidence descriptions. See Appendix A for the full inclusion criteria and Butler and colleagues (2020) for a complete description of the design of the AHRQ systematic review.

An important step in the AHRQ systematic review was to assess potentially eligible studies for risk of bias—the extent to which the study design and procedures are likely to have guarded against sources of bias that could affect the results. The tool used by the Minnesota EPC to assess risk of bias in studies of individual care interventions considers selection bias, attrition bias, detection bias, performance bias, and reporting bias (for the full tool, see Appendix A in Butler et al., 2020). Studies were classified as having a low, moderate, or high overall risk of bias based on the collective risk of bias across each of these five domains. For care delivery interventions, which were more likely than other interventions to be conducted in care settings and other real-life practice conditions with greater variability, the systematic review assessed only whether bias was over a certain threshold based on selection bias, level of attrition, and fidelity to the intervention. Studies identified as having low or moderate risk of bias were included in an *analytic set* on which the systematic review's analysis of strength of evidence was based. Studies identified as having a high risk of bias were included in the systematic review's *evidence maps*, which describe which interventions have been studied in the literature but were not included in the review's further analysis.

The final AHRQ systematic review has several strengths: (1) it is the product of a systematic and extensive effort to survey the body of literature and summarize the state of the evidence; (2) it has clear criteria for including and excluding studies were used; (3) it sheds light on the question of whether any interventions are supported by such conclusive and consistent evidence as to warrant an immediate recommendation for broad use without qualification or further study; and (4) it provides a helpful overview of the evidence landscape, including highlighting which interventions have been the subject of numerous studies, as well as challenges in the field, such as the large number of small-sample and pilot studies without corresponding larger or longer follow-on studies.

Limitations of the Approach and Existing Evidence

The AHRQ systematic review highlights significant challenges in the field. No interventions met the review's criteria for high-strength or moderate evidence of benefit, and only two types of intervention met the review's criteria for low-strength evidence of benefit. The ability to draw conclusions regarding the effectiveness of interventions in this domain was impeded by the small number of included studies for most categories of interventions, limitations in study design and execution, and variability across studies (e.g., in intervention implementation, comparison groups, outcomes measured, and study timing) that prohibited the pooling of data. Over time, standards for research are becoming more rigorous, but this progress is not yet fully reflected in the overall body of literature assessed in the AHRQ systematic review.

The AHRQ systematic review is a high-level assessment of the state of the science designed specifically to inform the question of which interventions, if any, are ready for broad dissemination and implementation. The AHRQ systematic review authors made decisions through this lens, including the exclusion of studies judged to be pilots, that inform the interpretation of the review findings and conclusions (see Chapter 5 for further discussion). Had the review targeted specific interventions in more depth and included research-setting efficacy studies without applying the lens of readiness for dissemination and implementation, the analysis and conclusions might have looked different.

Mixed results observed across RCTs may reflect heterogeneity in enrolled populations, settings, or other contextual factors. Given the wide range of needs, values, preferences, and desires of persons living with dementia, care partners, and caregivers, many interventions in this domain appropriately begin from the premise of individualization. It is also entirely expected that interventions will vary in effectiveness across different populations and in different settings. Furthermore, many factors beyond effectiveness that are critical for successful implementation, such as integration into workflow, may vary across settings, but these differences may be obscured as results are synthesized in a broad-scope systematic review. Given that these variations are inherently expected, and given the limitations in study design observed in many studies in this field, it is currently impossible to determine via a high-level systematic review of such a multifaceted situation whether an intervention is ineffective, whether it is effective but only for some people or in certain settings, or whether only certain of its elements are effective.

The systematic review is also necessarily limited to existing literature; it cannot synthesize evidence that does not yet exist, and it also reflects past research priorities. In the context of dementia care, this basic fact presents two particular challenges. First, while the situation is changing, the perspectives of persons living with dementia, care partners, and caregivers have historically not been central to identifying the needs, interventions, and outcomes to be studied by research (Gove et al., 2018). As a result, the studies evaluated in the systematic review often do not address the clinical significance of the findings, that is, whether the effect being demonstrated really matters to stakeholders. Moreover, interventions that target important outcomes for persons living with dementia, care partners, and caregivers may be absent from the existing literature. Second, racial and ethnic minorities have been significantly underrepresented in most dementia care studies (e.g., Dilworth-Anderson et al., 2020). Interventions that effectively address their needs may similarly be absent from the literature, or may be present in smaller studies that are not considered in the systematic review's analysis.

Lastly, it is important to recognize that the systematic review approach largely precluded consideration of evidence related to systems-based interventions. Examples of such interventions include the introduction of dementia care planning codes or dementia quality measures, or the effects of state or federal policy related to support for family caregivers or training for direct care workers, which do not lend themselves to assessment via an RCT.

Use of the GRADE Evidence to Decision (EtD) Framework and Supplemental Evidence

Consistent with its charge, the committee relied on the findings from the AHRQ systematic review to identify the interventions recommended for widespread dissemination and implementation with monitoring and evaluation, quality improvement, and information sharing. In addition to effectiveness, however, many factors need to be considered in determining whether broad implementation of an intervention is appropriate.

To inform its recommendation regarding dissemination and implementation, the committee applied the Grading of Recommendations Assessment, Development and Evaluation (GRADE) Evidence to Decision (EtD) framework to the two types of interventions identified in the systematic review as supported by low-strength evidence of benefit. The EtD framework can be applied to making and using clinical recommendations, coverage decisions, and health system and public health recommendations and decisions (Moberg et al., 2018). Factors taken into account in the EtD assessment can include the priority of the problem, how substantial the benefits and harms are, the certainty of the evidence, the value of the outcomes to stakeholders, how the intervention in question compares with others, resource requirements, cost-effectiveness relative to comparable options, the impact on health equity, the acceptability of the intervention to stakeholders, and the feasibility of implementation. For this assessment, the committee supplemented the AHRQ systematic review's analysis with additional evidence from published papers describing different adaptations and implementations of these two types of interventions. Some of these studies (e.g., studies with a single pre–posttest) used methodologies that did not meet the AHRQ systematic review's inclusion criteria. Nevertheless, as a complement to the studies included in the AHRQ systematic review, these studies provide such information as feasibility, equity, and resources required, which are important to inform decisions about implementation in the real world.

To guide research investments going forward and to extract the maximum value from the large body of interventions for which the evidence was determined to be insufficient, the committee sought to identify gaps in and opportunities to improve and expand the evidence base for dementia care interventions. As part of this assessment, the committee considered interventions for which there is some signal of benefit and that are unlikely to cause harm. A signal of benefit may be insufficient to recommend interventions for broad dissemination and implementation, which was the focus of the AHRQ systematic review and necessitates a high level of certainty in the evidence. However, the committee believed that a more holistic view of the available evidence—including input from persons living with dementia and their care partners and caregivers regarding their values, preferences, and needs—is appropriate to guide future research. Therefore, in addition to examining the AHRQ systematic review's intervention categories for potential signals of benefit, the committee considered such sources as stakeholder testimony during the committee's public information-gathering meetings, including testimony from persons living with dementia, care partners, and caregivers and representatives from advocacy organizations, professional associations, care systems, and payers; the Best Practice Caregiving database, which provides information from real-world implementation of interventions in practice settings (Benjamin Rose Institute on Aging and FCA, 2020a); and reports and presentations from the two National Research Summits on Care, Services, and Supports for Persons with Dementia and Their Caregivers (Gitlin and Maslow, 2018; Sferrazza, 2020). The committee's approach to assessing the evidence is described in greater detail in Chapter 5.

OTHER RELATED INITIATIVES

Reflecting the importance of its topic, this report falls within a broad set of initiatives aimed at advancing the development of and disseminating information about care, services, and supports for persons living with dementia and their care partners and caregivers. In addition to extensive research under way in academic settings, including at large dementia-focused centers, this section briefly mentions several of these initiatives. Additional research and nonresearch programs and initiatives relevant to improving dementia care, services, and supports are discussed in Chapter 4.

Two National Research Summits on Care, Services, and Supports for Persons with Dementia and Their Caregivers[2] in 2017 and 2020 con-

[2] The webpage for the National Research Summit can be accessed at https://aspe.hhs.gov/national-research-summit-care-services-and-supports-persons-dementia-and-their-caregivers (accessed January 28, 2021).

vened professionals and stakeholders from diverse backgrounds to identify evidence-based programs and research priorities that could improve the current state of care, services, and supports for persons living with dementia and caregivers (NIA, 2020). With a forward-looking focus aimed at driving future research and action, these summits have produced a number of recommendations regarding dementia care and research across 12 themes based on contributions from researchers, clinicians, and stakeholders, including persons living with dementia, care partners and caregivers, service providers, government programs, and payers (Gitlin and Maslow, 2018; Sferrazza, 2020).

Recognizing the need to accelerate and improve methods for testing and adoption of evidence-based interventions within health care systems, NIA also initiated and supports the IMbedded Pragmatic Alzheimer's disease and related dementias Clinical Trials (IMPACT) Collaboratory.[3] Established in 2019, the IMPACT Collaboratory is intended to build capacity for conducting pragmatic clinical trials of interventions embedded within health care systems by developing best methodological practices; supporting pragmatic clinical trials, including pilots, as well as training and dissemination of knowledge; supporting collaboration; and ensuring that research includes cultural tailoring and people from diverse and underrepresented backgrounds (NIA IMPACT Collaboratory, n.d.).

The Best Practice Caregiving database compiles evidence-based interventions for caregivers that have been implemented as a regular service of a community or health care organization.[4] The database includes information on the components, implementation, and effectiveness of more than 40 caregiver interventions (Benjamin Rose Institute on Aging and FCA, 2020b). In providing this information, Best Practice Caregiving aims to promote the broader uptake of these interventions by health and social service organizations (Benjamin Rose Institute on Aging, 2020).

A recently published report by the Lancet Commission, produced by an international group of dementia researchers and other experts and policy makers, highlights several interventions that have demonstrated evidence of improving outcomes for persons living with dementia and their care partners and caregivers. The Lancet Commission's findings prioritize evidence that is likely to have the greatest potential for impact in the global effort to find effective dementia care interventions (Livingston et al., 2020).

Finally, the National Academies is currently conducting a decadal survey to inform a research agenda for behavioral and social science research

[3] The webpage for the NIA IMPACT Collaboratory can be accessed at https://impactcollaboratory.org (accessed January 28, 2021).

[4] The webpage for the Best Practice Caregiving database can be accessed at https://bpc.caregiver.org/#searchPrograms (accessed January 28, 2021).

on AD/ADRD during the next decade (2020–2030). Drawing on extensive input from the scientific community and other stakeholders, the committee appointed to undertake that study has been asked to assess the role of the social and behavioral sciences in reducing the burden of AD/ADRD (NASEM, 2020).

REPORT ORGANIZATION

Following this introductory chapter, Chapter 2 outlines guiding principles for and core components of dementia care, services, and supports that recognize persons living with dementia as unique individuals and aim to support them, as well as their care partners and caregivers, in living well. Chapter 3 describes the complex systems in which dementia care, services, and supports are delivered. This chapter includes the committee's multilevel systems framework for care interventions for persons living with dementia and their care partners and caregivers. Chapter 4 outlines the committee's approach for evaluating the evidence on which interventions are ready for broad dissemination and implementation. This chapter includes a discussion of implementation science and stakeholder perspectives on making decisions about whether and how to implement interventions. Chapter 5 provides the committee's analysis of the available evidence and recommendations regarding the implementation of the two types of interventions for which the AHRQ systematic review found low-strength evidence of benefit—collaborative care models and REACH (Resources for Enhancing Alzheimer's Caregiver Health) II and its adaptations—with monitoring and evaluation, quality improvement, and information sharing. This chapter also provides additional assessment of the current state of the evidence, and identifies research gaps and opportunities. Finally, Chapter 6 presents a blueprint for future research, including an emphasis on addressing the needs and desires of persons living with dementia and their care partners and caregivers, cross-cutting methodological improvements for future studies that would enhance the strength of evidence in this field, prioritization of inclusive research, and a focus on assessing effectiveness in the real world.

REFERENCES

ASPE (Office of the Assistant Secretary for Planning and Evaluation). 2020. *National plans to address Alzheimer's disease*. https://aspe.hhs.gov/national-plans-address-alzheimers-disease (accessed January 15, 2021).

Benjamin Rose Institute on Aging. 2020. *About the project*. https://bpc.caregiver.org/#about (accessed September 2, 2020).

Benjamin Rose Institute on Aging and FCA (Family Caregiver Alliance). 2020a. *Best practice caregiving*. https://bpc.caregiver.org/#searchPrograms (accessed August 12, 2020).

Benjamin Rose Institute on Aging and FCA. 2020b. *Overview of the methodology.* https://bpc.caregiver.org/#methodology (accessed September 2, 2020).

Burgdorf, J., D. L. Roth, C. Riffin, and J. L. Wolff. 2019. Factors associated with receipt of training among caregivers of older adults. *JAMA Internal Medicine* 179(6):833–835.

Butler, M., J. E. Gaugler, K. M. C. Talley, H. I. Abdi, P. J. Desai, S. Duval, M. L. Forte, V. A. Nelson, W. Ng, J. M. Ouellette, E. Ratner, J. Saha, T. Shippee, B. L. Wagner, T. J. Wilt, and L. Yeshi. 2020. Care interventions for people living with dementia and their caregivers. *Comparative Effectiveness Review No. 231.* Rockville, MD: Agency for Healthcare Research and Quality. doi: 10.23970/AHRQEPCCER231.

Dilworth-Anderson, P., H. C. Hendrie, J. J. Manly, A. S. Khachaturian, and S. Fazio. 2008. Diagnosis and assessment of Alzheimer's disease in diverse populations. *Alzheimer's & Dementia* 4(4):305–309.

Dilworth-Anderson, P., H. Moon, and M. P. Aranda. 2020. Dementia caregiving research: Expanding and reframing the lens of diversity, inclusivity, and intersectionality. *Gerontologist* 60(5):797–805.

Fabius, C. D., J. L. Wolff, and J. D. Kasper. 2020. Race differences in characteristics and experiences of Black and white caregivers of older Americans. *The Gerontologist* 60(7):1244–1253.

Gianattasio, K. Z., C. Prather, M. M. Glymour, A. Ciarleglio, and M. C. Power. 2019. Racial disparities and temporal trends in dementia misdiagnosis risk in the United States. *Alzheimer's & Dementia* 5:891–898.

Gilsanz, P., M. M. Corrada, C. Kawas, E. R. Mayeda, M. M. Glymour, C. P. Quesenberry Jr., C. Lee, and R. A. Whitmer. 2019. Incidence of dementia after age 90 in a multiracial cohort. *Alzheimer's & Dementia* 15(4):497–505.

Gitlin, L. N., and N. Hodgson. 2018. *Better living with dementia: Implications for individuals, families, communities, and societies.* London, UK: Academic Press.

Gitlin, L. N., and K. Maslow. 2018. *National Research Summit on Care, Services, and Supports for Persons with Dementia and Their Caregivers: Report to the National Advisory Council on Alzheimer's Research, Care, and Services.* https://aspe.hhs.gov/system/files/pdf/259156/FinalReport.pdf (accessed September 1, 2020).

Gitlin, L. N., K. Marx, I. H. Stanley, and N. Hodgson. 2015. Translating evidence-based dementia caregiving interventions into practice: State-of-the-science and next steps. *Gerontologist* 55(2):210–226.

Gove, D., A. Diaz-Ponce, J. Georges, E. Moniz-Cook, G. Mountain, R. Chattat, L. Øksnebjerg, and the European Working Group of People with Dementia. 2018. Alzheimer Europe's position on involving people with dementia in research through PPI (patient and public involvement). *Aging & Mental Health* 22(6):723–729.

Han, A., J. Radel, J. M. McDowd, and D. Sabata. 2016. Perspectives of people with dementia about meaningful activities: A synthesis. *American Journal of Alzheimer's Disease & Other Dementias* 31(2):115–123.

Kelley, A. S., K. McGarry, R. Gorges, and J. S. Skinner. 2015. The burden of health care costs in the last 5 years of life. *Annals of Internal Medicine* 163(10):729–736.

Livingston, G., J. Huntley, A. Sommerlad, D. Ames, C. Ballard, S. Banerjee, C. Brayne, A. Burns, J. Cohen-Mansfield, C. Cooper, S. G. Costafreda, A. Dias, N. Fox, L. N. Gitlin, R. Howard, H. C. Kales, M. Kivimäki, E. B. Larson, A. Ogunniyi, V. Orgeta, K. Ritchie, K. Rockwood, E. L. Sampson, Q. Samus, L. S. Schneider, G. Selbæk, L. Teri, and N. Mukadam. 2020. Dementia prevention, intervention, and care: 2020 report of the Lancet Commission. *The Lancet* 396(10248):413–446.

Mayeda, E. R., M. M. Glymour, C. P. Quesenberry, and R. A. Whitmer. 2016. Inequalities in dementia incidence between six racial and ethnic groups over 14 years. *Alzheimer's & Dementia* 12(3):216–224.

Mitchell, S. L., V. Mor, P. L. Gozalo, J. L. Servadio, and J. M. Teno. 2016. Tube feeding in U.S. nursing home residents with advanced dementia, 2000-2014. *Journal of the American Medical Association* 316(7):769–770.

Mitchell, S. L., V. Mor, J. Harrison, and E. P. McCarthy. 2020. Embedded pragmatic trials in dementia care: Realizing the vision of the NIA IMPACT Collaboratory. *Journal of the American Geriatrics Society* 68(S2):S1–S7.

Moberg, J., A. D. Oxman, S. Rosenbaum, H. J. Schünemann, G. Guyatt, S. Flottorp, C. Glenton, S. Lewin, A. Morelli, G. Rada, P. Alonso-Coello, E. Akl, M. Gulmezoglu, R. A. Mustafa, J. Singh, E. von Elm, J. Vogel, J. Watine, and the GRADE Working Group. 2018. The GRADE Evidence to Decision (EtD) framework for health system and public health decisions. *Health Research Policy and Systems* 16(1):45.

NASEM (National Academies of Sciences, Engineering, and Medicine). 2016. *Families caring for an aging America.* Washington, DC: The National Academies Press.

NASEM. 2017. *Preventing cognitive decline and dementia: A way forward.* Washington, DC: The National Academies Press.

NASEM. 2018. *Considerations for the design of a systematic review of care interventions for individuals with dementia and their caregivers: Letter report.* Washington, DC: The National Academies Press.

NASEM. 2020. *Decadal survey of behavioral and social science research on Alzheimer's disease and Alzheimer's disease-related dementias.* https://www.nationalacademies.org/our-work/decadal-survey-of-behavioral-and-social-science-research-on-alzheimers-disease-and-alzheimers-disease-related-dementias (accessed October 22, 2020).

NIA (National Institute on Aging). 2020. *Summit virtual meeting series: 2020 National Research Summit on Care, Services, and Supports for Persons with Dementia and Their Caregivers.* https://www.nia.nih.gov/2020-dementia-care-summit#Registration (accessed September 1, 2020).

NIA IMPACT Collaboratory. n.d. *Overview.* https://impactcollaboratory.org/overview (accessed September 1, 2020).

Rivera-Hernandez, M., A. Kumar, G. Epstein-Lubow, and K. S. Thomas. 2019. Disparities in nursing home use and quality among African American, Hispanic, and white Medicare residents with Alzheimer's disease and related dementias. *Journal of Aging and Health* 31(7):1259–1277.

Roth, D. L., P. Dilworth-Anderson, J. Huang, A. L. Gross, and L. N. Gitlin. 2015. Positive aspects of family caregiving for dementia: Differential item functioning by race. *Journals of Gerontology: Series B* 70(6):813–819.

Sferrazza, C. 2020. *National Research Summit on Care, Services, and Supports for Persons with Dementia and Their Caregivers: Summit virtual meeting series—Summary report.* Bethesda, MD: National Institute on Aging.

Steenland, K., F. C. Goldstein, A. Levey, and W. Wharton. 2016. A meta-analysis of Alzheimer's disease incidence and prevalence comparing African-Americans and Caucasians. *Journal of Alzheimer's Disease* 50(1):71–76.

Willert, B., and K. L. Minnotte. 2019. Informal caregiving and strains: Exploring the impacts of gender, race, and income. *Applied Research in Quality of Life.* doi: 10.1007/s11482-019-09786-1.

2

MOVING TOWARD BETTER DEMENTIA CARE, SERVICES, AND SUPPORTS

Much progress has been made relative to how dementia care used to be provided. However, persons living with dementia and their care partners and caregivers are still struggling and are not living as well as they might. There are places where persons living with dementia and their care partners and caregivers are receiving and delivering high-quality care, supports, and services. But many individuals do not have access to such care, and, especially in disadvantaged communities, disparities are manifest in the care available and received.

The charge to this committee was to examine the evidence available to support decisions about policy and the broad dissemination and implementation of specific interventions, and to inform the relative prioritization of interventions that could be helpful but require resources, which are limited. To set the stage for the committee's response to that charge, this chapter explores fundamental concepts and principles that inform high-quality dementia care, services, and supports and takes stock of the journey toward providing better dementia care. The chapter ends with a set of guiding principles and core components that point to a better way to support persons living with dementia and their care partners and caregivers so they can thrive and live well.

LIVING WELL WITH DEMENTIA

The Experience of Persons Living with Dementia

Recent estimates place the number of people living with dementia in the United States somewhere between 3.7 and 5.8 million (Alzheimer's Association, 2020a; Nichols et al., 2019); globally, 37.8 to 51.0 million people are estimated to be living with dementia (Nichols et al., 2019). Dementia is a result of at least one disease—the most common being such neurodegenerative diseases as Alzheimer's disease, vascular disease, or Lewy body disease—that cause neurons to degenerate. In the past three decades, the United States, along with other wealthy countries, has experienced a steady decline in the risk of developing dementia (Livingston et al., 2020). This risk reduction has not been uniformly experienced, however, but instead relies on lifetime access to health care, particularly for cardiovascular disease; socioeconomic stability; and education (Livingston et al., 2020; Satizabal et al., 2016).

The symptoms of dementia can be categorized broadly as cognitive, functional, and behavioral, and may progressively worsen at different rates that are influenced by such factors as age of onset, sex, education, and history of hypertension (Haaksma et al., 2018; Tschanz et al., 2011). Improvement in the ability to detect and diagnose dementia earlier in its course led to the emergence of the diagnosis of mild cognitive impairment (MCI), a condition characterized by cognitive decline predominantly though not only in memory, but with normal functioning (Petersen et al., 2009). Common early symptoms of dementia include changes in memory; difficulties with attention, problem solving, and organization; and the emergence of anxiety (Gitlin and Hodgson, 2018). As the disease progresses, the person living with dementia may experience such symptoms as restlessness, anxiety, agitation, irritability, and aggressiveness. Along with these symptoms, the abilities of the person living with dementia to live independently and carry out activities of daily living decline. As a result, he or she relies more heavily on care partners or caregivers (Gitlin and Hodgson, 2018; NRC, 2010). In the late stage of dementia, the individual loses much of their ability to communicate verbally and needs a caregiver to meet daily needs (Gitlin and Hodgson, 2018) (see Figure 2-1). The average life expectancy after diagnosis for a person living with dementia due to Alzheimer's disease is around 4–6 years (Tom et al., 2015), though the average time between onset of symptoms and diagnosis is about 3 years (Thoits et al., 2018).

Reckoning with the early signs and symptoms of dementia can be a source of fear and distress for persons living with dementia, especially as they consider the implications for their independence (Gitlin and Hodgson, 2018). Moreover, the uncertainty of how the disease will affect them can lead to feelings of isolation, embarrassment, frustration, and confusion for persons living with dementia, as well as their family members and loved ones. Importantly, there is no singular experience of living with dementia. In fact, how individuals experience their own life with dementia is influenced by moderators of oppression and privilege, including race, ethnicity, gender expression, and class (Hulko, 2009). Individuals who face more

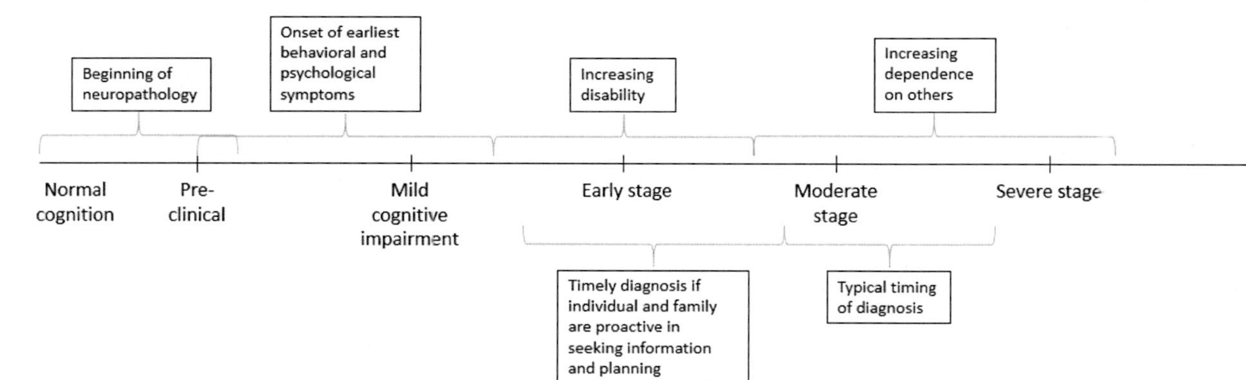

FIGURE 2-1 Timeline of typical disease progression in dementia.
SOURCE: Adapted from Gitlin and Hodgson, 2018.

marginalization based on these characteristics tend to view the memory deficits of dementia as less problematic, instead prioritizing the ability to carry out activities of daily living and instrumental activities of daily living as the measure of living well. Individuals with more privilege tend to have more social and emotional concerns, such as maintaining social roles, relationships, and independence, and generally have a more negative appraisal of their experience of living with dementia. Sexual and gender identity also intersect with the moderators mentioned above, such that LGBTQ individuals living with dementia are at increased risk of experiencing social isolation and poverty, especially if they belong to other marginalized groups (Alzheimer's Association and SAGE, 2018).

In the face of these challenges, however, action can be taken, such as adopting person-centered and strengths-based perspectives (both of which are discussed later in this chapter), to mitigate the fear and potential for loss of independence, identity, purpose, and relationships (Dementia Action Alliance and The Eden Alternative, 2020). Persons living with dementia are capable of leading meaningful and rewarding lives, finding enjoyment and pleasure from engaging in activities of interest, maintaining social relationships with others, and being connected to familiar environments and communities (Han et al., 2016). Social engagement, a quality relationship with a care partner or caregiver, and spirituality are factors that may further support a better quality of life for persons living with dementia (Martyr et al., 2018).

To live well, persons living with dementia need physical quality of life, social and emotional quality of life, and access to medical care and long-term services and supports (Black et al., 2013; Jennings et al., 2017). Medical care for persons living with dementia includes care specific to dementia, such as diagnosis, medications, and health education. It also includes care for other, comorbid conditions. Persons living with dementia frequently also live with one or more comorbid conditions, such as diabetes, cardiovascular disease, physical disabilities (e.g., limb loss, arthritis, sensory impairments), behavioral and psychiatric disorders (e.g., traumatic brain injuries, posttraumatic stress disorder [PTSD], bipolar disorder), and intellectual and developmental disabilities (e.g., Down syndrome, attention-deficit/hyperactivity disorder [ADHD], autism spectrum disorder). These conditions may affect the type and amount of care, services, and supports needed, as well as complicate both dementia care and care for other conditions.

Notably, however, much of what persons living with dementia need is support for functioning independently for as long as possible, living well in the world, and being able to participate in valued activities. In fact, some persons living with dementia prefer to remain living independently, especially in the early stages, and 13 percent live alone (Gould et al., 2015).

Long-term services and supports (LTSS) are provided to help people function as independently as possible for as long as possible in their own homes or in residential care settings (Thach and Wiener, 2018). LTSS may be delivered by care partners and caregivers (often family members and friends) or through formal care systems in the home and in formal residential settings, such as assisted living facilities and nursing homes. Persons living with dementia also need other services and supports, such as transportation and service coordination. As noted above, however, many persons living with dementia do not have access to or receive the care, supports, and services that would enable them to thrive. For example, one study found that 99 percent of persons living with dementia had at least one unmet need, with the average number of unmet needs being 7.7 (Black et al., 2013). In another large sample, every person living with dementia reported at least one unmet need, and the average number of unmet needs was 10.6 (Black et al., 2019). Ninety-seven percent of persons living with dementia reported unmet needs related to safety, including emergency planning; fall risk management; potential for abuse, neglect, and exploitation; and help with medication use and adherence. Eighty-three percent reported general health care needs not being met, including dental care, medical specialist care, incontinence care, and nutrition. Seventy-three percent reported unmet needs related to daily activities, including lack of meaningful activities, physical inactivity, and social isolation. Individuals who were racial and ethnic minorities, had lower educational attainment, had lower incomes, lived alone, and had mild dementia symptoms were more likely to have more unmet needs.

Because persons living with dementia are unique individuals—with their own values, including concerns related to privacy; needs; and preferences for services, supports, and medical care—the specific goals for and forms of care, services, and supports will depend on the individual. The recognition that persons living with dementia are still individuals is important to supporting them in leading lives with meaning, pleasure, and joy. Good care for persons living with dementia is about living a daily life, which is a deeply personal experience that draws on personal values and goals. Individuals have wide latitude to define what matters to them, what is fun, and what is boring. As a consequence of such cognitive problems as aphasia and impaired thought processing (Gitlin and Hodgson, 2018), however, persons with dementia may struggle to express their preferences, values, and goals, and their needs evolve over time.

Persons living with dementia have cognitive impairment that results in a disability, which is partially socially constructed by the way society views the disease and designs the living environment. To deal with their disabilities, persons living with dementia need accommodations that change how they interact with their environment, just as do persons with physical disabilities. Society has a legally recognized obligation to provide accommodations for persons with physical and mental disabilities.[1] For example, a person with paraplegia following spinal cord injury cannot enter a building via a flight of stairs. With the accommodation of a ramp or lift or the design of buildings without stairs, the impairment in leg mobility remains, but the ability to enter the building is supported. The recognition of persons living with dementia as experiencing a disability creates a parallel societal obligation to provide accommodations for that disability.

The disabilities experienced by persons living with dementia as a result of their cognitive impairments differ from the disabilities caused by physical impairments, and the accommodations they need differ accordingly. Their disabilities may be accommodated in part by such devices as a pill box, a list, a smartphone, and someday perhaps even a robot, especially as they transition from MCI to the mild stage of dementia and beyond. Because of the cognitive nature of their impairment, as well as the moral and creative dimensions of caregiving, these devices cannot fully substitute for a care partner or caregiver. A central premise of this report, then, is that the disabilities experienced by a person with dementia are generally accommodated by one or more people who help compensate for the person's cognitive impairments. These people—whether care partners, caregivers, or networks of people that change over time—represent an essential care component for persons living with dementia, who often rely on and want their involvement. They provide an accommodation for the cognitive nature of the disability by supporting another person's desires, needs, and preferences for living in the world and acting with intention to support and care for the person, particularly as he or she progresses to more advanced stages of the condition. People with other conditions, such as those who have had a stroke or persons with Parkinson's disease, may face similar challenges and similarly rely on care partners and caregivers; however, some persons living with dementia may not have any physical impairments but live with significant cognitive impairment.

The Role and Experience of Care Partners and Caregivers

Care partners and caregivers may be individuals who have an existing relationship with the person with dementia, such as close friends, a spouse, and other family members, or they may be direct care workers. A person with dementia may also rely on a combination of care partners and caregivers within their network of caregiving supports, which may change over time as the person's needs evolve. As of 2015, 21.6 million people in the United States were providing unpaid care for persons living with demen-

[1] Americans with Disabilities Act of 1990 (amended 2008), Public Law 101-336, 101st Cong. (July 26, 1990).

tia (Chi et al., 2019). One study estimates that only about one-quarter of persons living with dementia receive any care from a paid caregiver, and just 10 percent receive at least 20 hours of such care per week (Reckrey et al., 2020). Another study estimates that 63 percent of persons living with dementia receive only unpaid care, 5 percent receive only paid care, and 26 percent receive some combination of the two (Chi et al., 2019). While data are lacking on the number of persons living with dementia who do not receive any care from a care partner or caregiver, it is estimated that this is the case for 5 percent of persons living with dementia (Chi et al., 2019).

Care partners and caregivers engage in numerous roles and activities. They provide supports, services, programs, accommodations, or practices related to personal care (e.g., assisting with personal hygiene or getting dressed), and they help with medication management, paying bills, transportation, meal preparation, and health maintenance tasks (NASEM, 2016). They assist with activities, such as using transportation, cooking, managing finances, shopping, and cleaning a home, that allow a person to live independently in the community. In later stages of dementia, they assist with such self-care activities as transferring from a bed to a chair, bathing, getting dressed, feeding, and using the bathroom. The assistance they provide may be direct, or it may entail cueing the person to perform the activity. As caregivers assist with daily activities, they often take on the role of helping to make decisions; the two roles are often blended. For example, a caregiver may assist in preparing or even entirely providing dinner for a person with dementia, using person-centered techniques that might include some combination of such activities as asking the person what he or she would like to eat for dinner, doing the food shopping, and cooking the meal. Another role they may take on is attending medical and social service visits to help organize and deliver care to the person with dementia. The person living with dementia is considered the primary informant; for example, someone living with advanced symptoms of dementia can inform about experiencing pain through facial expressions. In the later stages of dementia, however, care partners and caregivers take on a greater role and often can provide useful contextual information, such as how often the pain occurs, under what circumstances, and with what associated symptoms. All of these roles ideally ensure that the person living with dementia lives a typical day that is safe and social and is engaged in meaningful activities. Sadly, however, this is not the case for many individuals throughout society, including persons living with dementia (Black et al., 2013).

Those who provide care for persons with dementia often experience positive aspects of caregiving, including a deeper appreciation for life, satisfaction with additional meaning in one's life, and strengthening of the relationship with the person living with dementia (NASEM, 2016; Roth et al., 2015). At the same time, however, care partners and caregivers also report stress and depression, loss of income, decreased well-being, and other consequences related to physical and mental health, family conflict, and social isolation (NASEM, 2016; Pinquart and Sörensen, 2003). Fully 97 percent of care partners and caregivers reported at least one unmet need, with an average of 4.6 unmet needs per caregiver (Black et al., 2013). Of these unmet needs, 89 percent were related to resource referrals, 85 percent to dementia education, and 45 percent to mental health care needs. The risk factors associated with a higher number of unmet needs for care partners and caregivers included being a racial minority and having lower educational attainment. Neither unpaid nor paid caregivers, such as home health aides or certified nursing assistants, receive adequate training and support for this challenging work (Burgdorf et al., 2019; NASEM, 2016).

Conceptions, perceptions, and experiences of the caregiving role vary significantly, including by culture, socioeconomic status, and educational level (Fabius et al., 2020; NASEM, 2016; Pinquart and Sörensen, 2005). Some care partners and caregivers may not see themselves as being in this role, instead perceiving their actions as an extension of existing familial roles, such as being a good spouse. In certain cultures, such as specific Latino cultures, the term caregiver is not used (Karlawish et al., 2011). If people who serve as care partners or caregivers do not see themselves in that role, they are unlikely to seek out and access services and supports even if available. Similarly, distrust of medical institutions, conceptions of the caregiving role as one of family responsibility, and feelings of shame have been described as factors that make African American and Asian American care partners and caregivers less likely to seek medical care and supports outside of the family (Apesoa-Varano et al., 2015; Dilworth-Anderson and Gibson, 2002).

A Complex and Dynamic Situation

As discussed above, dementia effectively joins at least two people: one the person living with dementia and the other a person or persons who provide care and support. While the focus is sometimes on a single care partner or caregiver—often a spouse or a child—persons living with dementia may receive support and help from combinations and networks of unpaid and paid caregivers, who may themselves be employed directly or associated with an agency, community organization, or residential facility. Together, persons living with dementia and their networks of care partners and caregivers need guidance and support that are essential to enable living in a rewarding way. They need education, guidance, and support to assist with activities of daily living and with planning and making decisions together, and they need medical and social services that help in organizing and delivering care. This guidance and support can ensure that both parties can enjoy a life that is safe, social, and engaged and that neither party experiences emotional, physical, or financial harms.

EVOLUTION OF THE UNDERSTANDING OF DEMENTIA AND DEMENTIA CARE

In the past 40 years, the United States has experienced two revolutions in thinking about persons living with dementia. What was once considered an extreme stage of normal aging of little medical importance became a consequence of diseases requiring medical attention—research, diagnosis, treatment, and care. What was once part of the duties of family members became more broadly recognized as a distinct role that has health and economic consequences.

Recognition of Dementia as a Medical Condition

Until the last two decades of the 20th century, late-life dementia was not widely recognized as the consequence of a disease. Older adults with dementia were described as having an extreme state of aging termed "senility," while adults with early-onset dementia were considered mentally ill (Ballenger, 2017). In fact, it was not until the 1940s and 1950s that the health care system began to take interest in the diagnosis and treatment of "the senile," abandoning earlier conceptions of dementia symptoms as an inevitable result of aging, which led to more widespread recognition of dementia as a public health issue beginning in the 1970s. Care for individuals with dementia was considered solely a private family matter, and the care of persons who lacked a family or whose family was unable to care for them became a matter of state welfare, typically provided in asylums and variations on facilities called "old age homes."

Figure 2-2 uses the results of a Google n-gram—a year-to-year summary of the frequency of a word's use in the English language—to illustrate the rapid redefinition and reframing of dementia. The figure shows how by the close of the 20th century, the term "senility" rapidly faded. In contrast, use of the terms "dementia" and "Alzheimer's disease" (the most common neurodegenerative disease thought to cause dementia) increased. Of late, the language has been further nuanced to truly distinguish the person from the disease and the illness experience, as exemplified by this report's use of the term "a person living with dementia." While most care continues to be delivered solely by family caregivers, there is now greater recognition of dementia care, services, and supports as a societal concern and responsibility, as described in greater detail below.

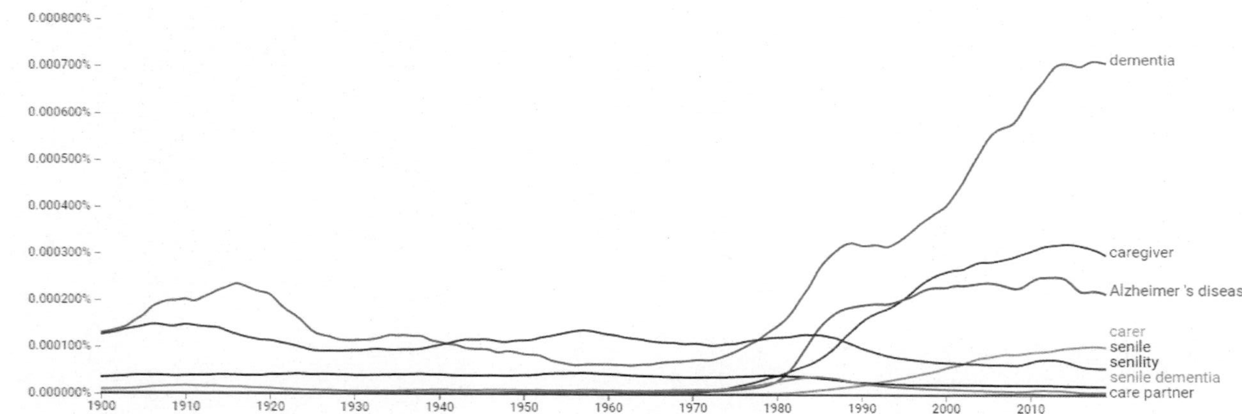

FIGURE 2-2 Google n-gram, a year-to-year summary of the frequency of a word's use in books in the English language from 1900 to 2019, for key terms related to dementia and dementia care.
SOURCE: Google Books Ngram Viewer.

Increasing Recognition of the Role and Consequences of Caregiving

Prior to the 1970s, the term "caregiver" was rarely used in the health, social service, or medical care literature. Figure 2-2 illustrates the sudden appearance and rapid rise of this term beginning in the 1980s. As noted above, prior to that time, caregiving was not recognized as distinct from other family roles. People did not self-identify as caregivers, attend support groups, or receive other supports and services designed for caregivers. A paid caregiver was variously referred to as a nurse, aide, or maid.

Starting in the late 1970s this situation began to change. The term "caregiver" (as well as such variations as "carer" and "caretaker") appeared abruptly (Brody, 1981; Shanas, 1979). Use of the term, which is not specific to dementia, grew rapidly. By the 1980s, the Alzheimer's Association, a national self-help organization, was offering support groups and training for caregivers (Alzheimer's Association, 2020b). Its first public service announcement, delivered in 1990 by the eminent journalist Walter Cronkite, stated: "Today, there are at least 4 million victims of Alzheimer's disease. But for almost every one of those victims, there is another, a husband or wife ... a son or daughter ... whose entire life changes with the demands of caregiving" (Alzheimer's Association, 1990). Such a statement would not have been heard in 1980.

Recognition of the role of the caregiver has been critical to improving dementia care. Caregiving is now recognized as part of the experience of dementia, such that the hours spent caregiving are used as facts and figures to describe the disease. In 2015, for example, a person living with dementia received an average of 127 hours of assistance per month from one or more unpaid caregivers (Chi et al., 2019), and it is estimated that this unpaid caregiving had an annual monetary value of \$50–\$106 billion as of 2010 (Hurd et al., 2013). This figure includes the cost of caregivers' lost wages and the value of their labor in providing care; another estimate that considers lost wages and indirect costs to caregivers' well-being places the cost of just the unpaid care provided by daughters to mothers at \$277 billion (Coe et al., 2018).

These figures are critical to understanding the size and scope of the dementia experience. When the hours devoted to caregiving are seen as work, they can be assigned a wage, and the wages of caregiving add up to nearly half of the costs of dementia in the United States (Hurd et al., 2013). Put another way, a substantial portion of the multi-billion-dollar cost of dementia to the nation consists of lost wages and other opportunity costs due to providing care instead of working in the "traditional" labor force. The average lifetime cost of dementia from time of diagnosis is \$321,780, with families assuming 70 percent (\$225,140) of this cost (Jutkowitz et al., 2017).

Moving Toward Person-Centered and Strengths-Based Approaches

Person-centered care—care that responds to the needs and preferences of the individual—has been increasing as a priority in health care over the past few decades (IOM, 2001). Increased adoption of person-centered care is also a growing focus in nursing home care and LTSS, as exemplified by Congress's call in the Patient Protection and Affordable Care Act of 2010 for the secretary of health and human services to develop regulations to ensure the delivery of patient-centered care in home- and community-based LTSS.[2] Person-centered care incorporates an understanding of an individual's culture and the challenges faced by members of that culture as well as their strengths, but is not restricted to cultural competence, recognizing that individuals within a culture also differ from one another (Epner and Baile, 2012).

Strengths-based approaches are a component of person-centered care that involves assessing and building on individuals' strengths, abilities, and available resources to promote their well-being and growth (McGovern, 2015; Moyle, 2014). In dementia care, adopting a strengths-based approach requires a focus on the present and on what abilities remain rather than what has been lost (Dementia Action Alliance and The Eden Alternative, 2020; McGovern, 2015). For example, tasks can be divided into smaller components that allow persons living with dementia to focus on their strengths, as well as create opportunities for growth and development of other capabilities (Dementia Action Alliance and The Eden Alternative, 2020). Importantly, an individual's abilities, interests, and strengths will change over time, and care partners and caregivers need to be flexible to respond to those changes so the person living with dementia is empowered to grow to the fullest extent possible. For example, an individual interested in music and the arts might be provided opportunities to actively make art and music in the earlier stages of dementia, and transition to spending time at museums or concerts with loved ones as symptoms progress. Strengths-based assessments can help identify an individual's emotional and behavioral skills, competencies, and characteristics in order to build on these strengths (Moyle, 2014). A strengths-based approach can empower persons living with dementia with the decision-making ability to determine the level of assistance needed while supporting the ability of care partners and caregivers to provide appropriate care (Dementia Action Alliance and The Eden Alternative, 2020). Indeed, the ways in which care partners and caregivers express their experiences, such as personal growth, the development of strengths, and a closer relationship with the person living with dementia, often accord with strengths-based perspectives (Peacock et al., 2010).

---

[2] 42 USC 1396n note. Regulations. Oversight and Assessment of the Administration of Home and Community-based Services.

Person-centered and strengths-based approaches may help shift the focus from the diagnosis of dementia to the person living with dementia and the accommodations and lifestyle changes that can be adopted to support the person in leading a rewarding life.

Policy Implications

The recognition of dementia as a consequence of disease and of someone who cares for a person with dementia as a care partner or caregiver has notable policy implications. It argues for the responsibility of the care system—including medical care; LTSS; and other social services and supports, such as respite care, adult day activity programs, and transportation—to provide care and support for persons living with dementia and their care partners and caregivers. One major challenge is that there is recognition of a workforce shortage for geriatric practitioners generally (IOM, 2008), as well as for direct care providers, such as nurse aides and home health aides, who tend to deliver care in long-term care facilities or in an individual's home (Scales, 2020). As the number of Americans over age 65 diagnosed with Alzheimer's disease and other dementias is expected to grow, so, too, is the demand for direct care workers (PHI, 2020). Yet, projections show that the shortages in the direct care workforce will increase from 2018 to 2028 (PHI, 2020), compounded by a high rate of turnover in the field (Scales, 2020). Thus, there is a need to improve recruitment and retention in this field (IOM, 2008).

This increased recognition of societal responsibility is reflected in the U.S. National Alzheimer's Plan, initiated in 2012 through the National Alzheimer's Project Act (NAPA). The first goal of this plan is to prevent and effectively treat Alzheimer's disease by 2025 (ASPE, 2020). However, recognizing that persons living with dementia, care partners, and caregivers need support now and for the foreseeable future, the second and third goals are to optimize the quality and efficiency of care, and to expand supports for people living with Alzheimer's disease and their families. Curing and caring are appropriately viewed as in harmony for dementia, as they are for other conditions, such as cancer and cardiovascular disease.[3]

Supporting the goals of the National Alzheimer's Plan, the National Research Summit on Care, Services, and Supports for Persons with Dementia and Their Caregivers was convened in 2017 by the National

[3] For example, the cancer centers funded by the National Cancer Institute (NCI) recognize the need to harmonize cures and care. The criteria for a Cancer Center Support Grant include the expectation that the NCI-designated cancer center director will align research and care missions, as described in the Request for Applications at https://grants.nih.gov/grants/guide/pa-files/par-20-043.html (accessed January 28, 2021).

Advisory Panel on Alzheimer's Research, Care, and Services, and again in 2020 by the National Institute on Aging (NIA). These summits bring stakeholders together to discuss evidence-based programs, strategies, and approaches for improving dementia care, services, and supports, as well as to identify research gaps and opportunities in the field (NIA, 2020). Consistent with the movement toward person-centered approaches described above, the summits incorporate and highlight voices of persons living with dementia, care partners, and caregivers, as well as researchers, care organizations, and other stakeholders. In addition, advocacy organizations, such as the Alzheimer's Association, are collaborating with various partners to carry out specific actions of the National Alzheimer's Plan (HHS, 2019), and other organizations, such as the National Alliance for Caregiving and the Alzheimer's Foundation of America, have provided guidance on how to implement the plan at the state and local levels (National Alliance for Caregiving and Alzheimer's Foundation of America, 2014). Also involved in advocacy for policy change are such groups as The Alzheimer's Impact Movement and Activists Against Alzheimer's, the advocacy affiliates of the Alzheimer's Association and UsAgainstAlzheimer's, respectively, which bring together volunteers who promote federal and state policy regarding dementia research and care (Alzheimer's Impact Movement, n.d.; UsAgainstAlzheimer's, 2020).

GUIDING PRINCIPLES AND CORE COMPONENTS OF DEMENTIA CARE, SERVICES, AND SUPPORTS

The concepts outlined above provide the basis for a set of guiding principles for dementia care, services, and supports (see Box 2-1). In addition, various core components of dementia care services and supports have been identified (see Box 2-2). Together, these guiding principles and core components reflect shared community values that include principles of good/ethical care, standards of care, justice, and human dignity and thriving.

The lack of evidence available to answer the questions posed in the committee's charge (see Box 1-1 in Chapter 1), as detailed in subsequent chapters, does not call these fundamental principles or core components into question. Rather, it points to the need for additional research and programmatic assessment to address the gaps in information about specific interventions. In the interim, these guiding principles and core components can be used immediately by organizations, agencies, communities, and individuals to guide their actions toward improving dementia care, supports, and services. Given the critical shortcomings that now exist, if persons living with dementia and their care partners and caregivers had access to care, services, and supports guided by these principles and including these components, this would represent a significant advance.

BOX 2-1
Guiding Principles for Dementia Care, Services, and Supports

The following principles can help guide care, services, and supports for persons living with dementia and their care partners and caregivers. Unfortunately, their application is currently limited.

Person-centeredness: Recognition of persons living with dementia as individuals with their own goals, desires, interests, and abilities.

Promotion of well-being: The use of social, behavioral, and environmental interventions that address the needs of persons living with dementia, care partners, and caregivers holistically to enhance well-being.

Respect and dignity: Attention to each person's particular needs and values, including privacy, which may be achieved by following models for eliciting preferences and values, such as values elicitation, supported decision making, shared decision making, respect for dissent, or seeking either assent or informed consent.

Justice: Treating people with equal need equally, such that, for example, all critically ill persons receive critical care, all expectant mothers receive prenatal care, and the dying receive palliative care. By extension, all persons living with dementia, care partners, and caregivers have access to and can receive care, supports, and services that enable them to live well.

Racial, ethnic, sexual, cultural, and linguistic inclusivity: The availability of racially, ethnically, sexually, culturally, and linguistically appropriate services to all who may need them, especially underserved and underrepresented populations, such as racial and ethnic minorities and LGBTQ individuals.

Accessibility and affordability: Care, services, and supports for persons living with dementia, care partners, and caregivers that do not impose an unmanageable financial burden on individuals or their families and are available and accessible to all who may need them, including in rural communities.

SOURCES: Fazio et al., 2018; Livingston et al., 2020; NQF, 2014.

Furthermore, there are many activities, such as listening to music and dancing, that provide pleasure for many people living with or without dementia and likely have little potential harm apart from opportunity and financial costs. At the individual or family level, persons living with dementia and their care partners and caregivers may want to experiment with these types of activities, tailored to their own interests, to see what works for them, knowing this may change as the person's condition progresses.

BOX 2-2
Core Components of Care, Services, and Supports for Persons Living with Dementia, Care Partners, and Caregivers

Several existing frameworks describe core components of ideal dementia care, supports, and services. Common elements of these frameworks are synthesized below to highlight the core components that promote the well-being of persons living with dementia, care partners, and caregivers. These components are ideally designed with participation of the individuals involved and managed throughout the course of the condition, and need to be adjusted according to the many changes experienced by persons living with dementia, care partners, and caregivers.

Detection and diagnosis: Early detection and diagnosis of dementia is important so that persons living with dementia and their care partners and caregivers can receive the care, services, and supports they need. Notably, some people with symptoms may not want to seek detection, diagnosis, or services because of such factors as cultural norms and practices and concerns about loss of autonomy, privacy, relationships, or jobs. Providers therefore need to recognize the signs and symptoms of cognitive impairment and listen to the associated concerns expressed by individuals and family members.

Assessment of symptoms to inform planning and deliver care: The cognitive, functional, behavioral, and psychological status of the person living with dementia and the psychological status of the care partner or caregiver need to be assessed regularly. Those assessments are used to monitor the well-being of the person living with dementia and the care partner or caregiver and to provide education, problem solving, skill building, resources, and referrals as needs evolve. This includes planning for financial and legal matters and potential problems that can occur, such as ways to mitigate errors in financial management and prevent fraud or exploitation.

Information and education: Starting at the time of diagnosis, persons living with dementia, care partners, and caregivers benefit when clinicians provide clear information about the disease and offer additional educational resources and referrals. The provision of information on options for care, services, and supports is also crucial as the condition progresses, and should be responsive to evolving needs.

Medical management: Providers need to deliver holistic, person-centered medical care that prioritizes nonpharmacological interventions while including pharmacological interventions when appropriate. Discussions between clinicians and persons living with dementia, care partners, and caregivers can serve to develop a shared vision for care, track the progression of symptoms, and ensure the management of comorbidities.

Support in activities of daily living: Support in these activities needs to respect the abilities and preferences of the individual person living with dementia.

Support for care partners and caregivers: Recognizing and supporting the essential role of care partners and caregivers, as well as their unique challenges and needs, is important to their health, financial security, and well-being. This component encompasses referrals to supports and services.

Communication and collaboration: Well-documented information about the diagnosis, treatment, goals, and preferences of the person living with dementia, related to both dementia and any comorbidities, needs to be available to all those involved in the provision of services and care and to follow the person living with dementia during care transitions. Safe and responsive care requires that services and health care be provided through an interdisciplinary staff whose members communicate regularly and share information.

Coordination of medical care, long-term services and supports, and community-based services and supports: Quality dementia care combines medical care with community-based services and supports to provide a continuum of services that meet the complex needs and desires of persons living with dementia, care partners, and caregivers. Medical care and long-term services and supports also need to be coordinated in residential settings, including nursing homes, where residents with dementia commonly have serious comorbidities.

Supportive and safe environment: Physical spaces that ensure the safety of persons living with dementia, care partners, and caregivers are essential. Ideally, these spaces will provide opportunities for meaningful engagement and self-determination, and foster relationships between providers and persons living with dementia, care partners, and caregivers that promote dignity and respect.

Advance care planning and end-of-life care: Early discussions between providers and a person living with dementia and his or her family regarding the goals and desires of the person living with dementia are important to ensure respect for that person. Planning should continue throughout the disease's progression, with increasing dependence on the primary caregiver to communicate the goals and values of the person living with dementia when the person can no longer participate in this process. Given the unpredictable nature of dementia, initiation of palliative care is based on need and preferences, not prognosis.

SOURCES: Benjamin Rose Institute on Aging and FCA, 2020; Boustani et al., 2019; Fazio et al., 2018; Livingston et al., 2020; NASEM, 2016; NQF, 2014; Zimmerman et al., 2011.

REFERENCES

Alzheimer's Association. 1990. 4 million. In *Walter Cronkite Papers, 1932–2014*. Austin: Dolph Briscoe Center for American History at the University of Texas.

Alzheimer's Association. 2020a. 2020 Alzheimer's disease facts and figures. *Alzheimer's & Dementia* 16(3):391–460.

Alzheimer's Association. 2020b. *Our story*. https://www.alz.org/about/our_story (accessed November 23, 2020).

Alzheimer's Association and SAGE. 2018. *Issues brief: LGBT and dementia*. https://www.alz.org/media/documents/lgbt-dementia-issues-brief.pdf (accessed December 22, 2020).

Alzheimer's Impact Movement. n.d. *About the Alzheimer's impact movement*. https://alzimpact.org/about (accessed November 11, 2020).

Apesoa-Varano, E. C., Y. Tang-Feldman, S. C. Reinhard, R. Choula, and H. M. Young. 2015. Multi-cultural caregiving and caregiver interventions: A look back and a call for future action. *Generations* 39(4):39–48.

ASPE (Office of the Assistant Secretary for Planning and Evaluation). 2020. *National plans to address Alzheimer's disease*. https://aspe.hhs.gov/national-plans-address-alzheimers-disease (accessed January 15, 2021).

Ballenger, J. F. 2017. Framing confusion: Dementia, society, and history. *American Medical Association Journal of Ethics* 19(7):713–719.

Benjamin Rose Institute on Aging and FCA (Family Caregiver Alliance). 2020. *Best practice caregiving*. https://bpc.caregiver.org/#searchPrograms (accessed August 12, 2020).

Black, B. S., D. Johnston, P. V. Rabins, A. Morrison, C. Lyketsos, and Q. M. Samus. 2013. Unmet needs of community-residing persons with dementia and their informal caregivers: Findings from the maximizing independence at home study. *Journal of the American Geriatrics Society* 61(12):2087–2095.

Black, B. S., D. Johnston, J. Leoutsakos, M. Reuland, J. Kelly, H. Amjad, K. Davis, A. Willink, D. Sloan, C. Lyketsos, and Q. M. Samus. 2019. Unmet needs in community-living persons with dementia are common, often non-medical and related to patient and caregiver characteristics. *International Psychogeriatrics* 31(11):1643–1654.

Boustani, M., C. A. Alder, C. A. Solid, and D. Reuben. 2019. An alternative payment model to support widespread use of collaborative dementia care models. *Health Affairs* 38(1):54–59.

Brody, E. M. 1981. "Women in the middle" and family help to older people. *Gerontologist* 21(5):471–480.

Burgdorf, J., D. L. Roth, C. Riffin, and J. L. Wolff. 2019. Factors associated with receipt of training among caregivers of older adults. *JAMA Internal Medicine* 179(6):833–835.

Chi, W., E. Graf, L. Hughes, J. Hastie, G. Khatutsky, S. B. Shuman, E. A. Jessup, S. Karon, and H. Lamont. 2019. *Community-dwelling older adults with dementia and their caregivers: Key indicators from the national health and aging trends study.* Washington, DC: Office of the Assistant Secretary for Planning and Evaluation.

Coe, N. B., M. M. Skira, and E. B. Larson. 2018. A comprehensive measure of the costs of caring for a parent: Differences according to functional status. *Journal of the American Geriatrics Society* 66(10):2003–2008.

Dementia Action Alliance and The Eden Alternative. 2020. *Practice guide for assisted living communities: Person- and relationship-centered dementia support.* https://www.edenalt-evolve.org/courses/raising-the-bar-practice-guide-assisted-living (accessed January 20, 2021).

Dilworth-Anderson, P., and B. E. Gibson. 2002. The cultural influence of values, norms, meanings, and perceptions in understanding dementia in ethnic minorities. *Alzheimer's Disease & Associated Disorders* 16:S56–S63.

Epner, D. E., and W. F. Baile. 2012. Patient-centered care: The key to cultural competence. *Annals of Oncology* 23(Suppl 3):33–42.

Fabius, C. D., J. L. Wolff, and J. D. Kasper. 2020. Race differences in characteristics and experiences of black and white caregivers of older americans. *Gerontologist* 60(7):1244–1253.

Fazio, S., D. Pace, K. Maslow, S. Zimmerman, and B. Kallmyer. 2018. Alzheimer's Association dementia care practice recommendations. *Gerontologist* 58(Suppl 1):S1–S9.

Gitlin, L. N., and N. Hodgson. 2018. *Better living with dementia: Implications for individuals, families, communities, and societies*. London, UK: Academic Press.

Gould, E., K. Maslow, M. Lepore, L. Bercaw, J. Leopold, B. Lyda-McDonald, M. Ignaczak, P. Yuen, and J. M. Wiener. 2015. *Identifying and meeting the needs of individuals with dementia who live alone*. Washington, DC: RTI International.

Haaksma, M. L., A. Calderón-Larrañaga, M. G. M. Olde Rikkert, R. J. F. Melis, and J. S. Leoutsakos. 2018. Cognitive and functional progression in Alzheimer disease: A prediction model of latent classes. *International Journal of Geriatric Psychiatry* 33(8):1057–1064.

Han, A., J. Radel, J. M. McDowd, and D. Sabata. 2016. Perspectives of people with dementia about meaningful activities: A synthesis. *American Journal of Alzheimer's Disease & Other Dementias* 31(2):115–123.

HHS (U.S. Department of Health and Human Services). 2019. *National plan to address Alzheimer's disease: 2019 update*. https://aspe.hhs.gov/system/files/pdf/262601/NatlPlan2019.pdf (accessed October 1, 2020).

Hulko, W. 2009. From "not a big deal" to "hellish": Experiences of older people with dementia. *Journal of Aging Studies* 23(3):131–144.

Hurd, M. D., P. Martorell, A. Delavande, K. J. Mullen, and K. M. Langa. 2013. Monetary costs of dementia in the United States. *New England Journal of Medicine* 368(14):1326–1334.

IOM (Institute of Medicine). 2001. *Crossing the quality chasm: A new health system for the 21st century*. Washington, DC: National Academy Press.

IOM. 2008. *Retooling for an aging America: Building the health care workforce*. Washington, DC: The National Academies Press.

Jennings, L. A., A. Palimaru, M. G. Corona, X. E. Cagigas, K. D. Ramirez, T. Zhao, R. D. Hays, N. S. Wenger, and D. B. Reuben. 2017. Patient and caregiver goals for dementia care. *Quality of Life Research* 26(3):685–693.

Jutkowitz, E., R. L. Kane, J. E. Gaugler, R. F. MacLehose, B. Dowd, and K. M. Kuntz. 2017. Societal and family lifetime cost of dementia: Implications for policy. *Journal of the American Geriatrics Society* 65(10):2169–2175.

Karlawish, J., F. K. Barg, D. Augsburger, J. Beaver, A. Ferguson, and J. Nunez. 2011. What Latino Puerto Ricans and non-Latinos say when they talk about Alzheimer's disease. *Alzheimer's & Dementia* 7(2):161–170.

Livingston, G., J. Huntley, A. Sommerlad, D. Ames, C. Ballard, S. Banerjee, C. Brayne, A. Burns, J. Cohen-Mansfield, C. Cooper, S. G. Costafreda, A. Dias, N. Fox, L. N. Gitlin, R. Howard, H. C. Kales, M. Kivimäki, E. B. Larson, A. Ogunniyi, V. Orgeta, K. Ritchie, K. Rockwood, E. L. Sampson, Q. Samus, L. S. Schneider, G. Selbæk, L. Teri, and N. Mukadam. 2020. Dementia prevention, intervention, and care: 2020 report of the Lancet Commission. *The Lancet* 396(10248):413–446.

Martyr, A., S. M. Nelis, C. Quinn, Y.-T. Wu, R. A. Lamont, C. Henderson, R. Clarke, J. V. Hindle, J. M. Thom, I. R. Jones, R. G. Morris, J. M. Rusted, C. R. Victor, and L. Clare. 2018. Living well with dementia: A systematic review and correlational meta-analysis of factors associated with quality of life, well-being and life satisfaction in people with dementia. *Psychological Medicine* 48(13):2130–2139.

McGovern, J. 2015. Living better with dementia: Strengths-based social work practice and dementia care. *Social Work in Health Care* 54(5):408–421.

Moyle, W. 2014. Principles of strengths-based care and other nursing models. In *Care of older adults: A strengths-based approach*, edited by W. Moyle, D. Parker, and M. Bramble. Port Melbourne, Australia: Cambridge University Press.

NASEM (National Academies of Sciences, Engineering, and Medicine). 2016. *Families caring for an aging America*. Washington, DC: The National Academies Press.

National Alliance for Caregiving and Alzheimer's Foundation of America. 2014. *From plan to practice: Implementing the national Alzheimer's plan in your state*. https://www.caregiving.org/creating-an-alzheimers-plan-for-your-state (accessed January 20, 2021).

NIA (National Institute on Aging). 2020. *Summit virtual meeting series: 2020 National Research Summit on Care, Services, and Supports for Persons with Dementia and Their Caregivers*. https://www.nia.nih.gov/2020-dementia-care-summit#Registration (accessed September 1, 2020).

Nichols, E., C. E. I. Szoeke, S. E. Vollset, N. Abbasi, F. Abd-Allah, J. Abdela, M. T. E. Aichour, R. O. Akinyemi, F. Alahdab, S. W. Asgedom, A. Awasthi, S. L. Barker-Collo, B. T. Baune, Y. Béjot, A. B. Belachew, D. A. Bennett, B. Biadgo, A. Bijani, M. S. Bin Sayeed, C. Brayne, D. O. Carpenter, F. Carvalho, F. Catalá-López, E. Cerin, J.-Y. J. Choi, A. K. Dang, M. G. Degefa, S. Djalalinia, M. Dubey, E. E. Duken, D. Edvardsson, M. Endres, S. Eskandarieh, A. Faro, F. Farzadfar, S.-M. Fereshtehnejad, E. Fernandes, I. Filip, F. Fischer, A. K. Gebre, D. Geremew, M. Ghasemi-Kasman, E. V. Gnedovskaya, R. Gupta, V. Hachinski, T. B. Hagos, S. Hamidi, G. J. Hankey, J. M. Haro, S. I. Hay, S. S. N. Irvani, R. P. Jha, J. B. Jonas, R. Kalani, A. Karch, A. Kasaeian, Y. S. Khader, I. A. Khalil, E. A. Khan, T. Khanna, T. A. M. Khoja, J. Khubchandani, A. Kisa, K. Kissimova-Skarbek, M. Kivimäki, A. Koyanagi, K. J. Krohn, G. Logroscino, S. Lorkowski, M. Majdan, R. Malekzadeh, W. März, J. Massano, G. Mengistu, A. Meretoja, M. Mohammadi, M. Mohammadi-Khanaposhtani, A. H. Mokdad, S. Mondello, G. Moradi, G. Nagel, M. Naghavi, G. Naik, L. H. Nguyen, T. H. Nguyen, Y. L. Nirayo, M. R. Nixon, R. Ofori-Asenso, F. A. Ogbo, A. T. Olagunju, M. O. Owolabi, S. Panda-Jonas, V. M. d. A. Passos, D. M. Pereira, G. D. Pinilla-Monsalve, M. A. Piradov, C. D. Pond, H. Poustchi, M. Qorbani, A. Radfar, R. C. Reiner, Jr., S. R. Robinson, G. Roshandel, A. Rostami, T. C. Russ, P. S. Sachdev, H. Safari, S. Safiri, R. Sahathevan, Y. Salimi, M. Satpathy, M. Sawhney, M. Saylan, S. G. Sepanlou, A. Shafieesabet, M. A. Shaikh, M. A. Sahraian, M. Shigematsu, R. Shiri, I. Shiue, J. P. Silva, M. Smith, S. Sobhani, D. J. Stein, R. Tabarés-Seisdedos, M. R. Tovani-Palone, B. X. Tran, T. T. Tran, A. T. Tsegay, I. Ullah, N. Venketasubramanian, V. Vlassov, Y.-P. Wang, J. Weiss, R. Westerman, T. Wijeratne, G. M. A. Wyper, Y. Yano, E. M. Yimer, N. Yonemoto, M. Yousefifard, Z. Zaidi, Z. Zare, T. Vos, V. L. Feigin, and C. J. L. Murray. 2019. Global, regional, and national burden of Alzheimer's disease and other dementias, 1990-2016: A systematic analysis for the global burden of disease study 2016. *The Lancet Neurology* 18(1):88–106.

NQF (National Quality Forum). 2014. *Priority setting for healthcare performance measurement: Addressing performance measure gaps for dementia, including Alzheimer's disease*. http://www.qualityforum.org/priority_setting_for_healthcare_performance_measurement_alzheimers_disease.aspx (accessed September 4, 2020).

NRC (National Research Council). 2010. *The role of human factors in home health care: Workshop summary*. Washington, DC: The National Academies Press.

Peacock, S., D. Forbes, M. Markle-Reid, P. Hawranik, D. Morgan, L. Jansen, B. D. Leipert, and S. R. Henderson. 2010. The positive aspects of the caregiving journey with dementia: Using a strengths-based perspective to reveal opportunities. *Journal of Applied Gerontology* 29(5):640–659.

Petersen, R. C., R. O. Roberts, D. S. Knopman, B. F. Boeve, Y. E. Geda, R. J. Ivnik, G. E. Smith, and C. R. Jack, Jr. 2009. Mild cognitive impairment: Ten years later. *Archives of Neurology* 66(12):1447–1455.

PHI. 2020. *Direct care workers in the United States: Key facts.* New York: PHI.

Pinquart, M., and S. Sörensen. 2003. Differences between caregivers and noncaregivers in psychological health and physical health: A meta-analysis. *Psychology and Aging* 18(2):250–267.

Pinquart, M., and S. Sörensen. 2005. Ethnic differences in stressors, resources, and psychological outcomes of family caregiving: A meta-analysis. *Gerontologist* 45(1):90–106.

Reckrey, J. M., R. S. Morrison, K. Boerner, S. L. Szanton, E. Bollens-Lund, B. Leff, and K. A. Ornstein. 2020. Living in the community with dementia: Who receives paid care? *Journal of the American Geriatrics Society* 68(1):186–191.

Roth, D. L., P. Dilworth-Anderson, J. Huang, A. L. Gross, and L. N. Gitlin. 2015. Positive aspects of family caregiving for dementia: Differential item functioning by race. *Journals of Gerontology: Series B* 70(6):813–819.

Satizabal, C. L., A. S. Beiser, V. Chouraki, G. Chêne, C. Dufouil, and S. Seshadri. 2016. Incidence of dementia over three decades in the Framingham Heart Study. *New England Journal of Medicine* 374(6):523–532.

Scales, K. 2020. *It's time to care: A detailed profile of America's direct care workforce.* New York: PHI.

Shanas, E. 1979. The family as a social support system in old age. *Gerontologist* 19(2):169–174.

Thach, N. T., and J. M. Wiener. 2018. *An overview of long-term services and supports and Medicaid: Final report.* Washington, DC: U.S. Department of Health and Human Services.

Thoits, T., A. Dutkiewicz, S. Raguckas, M. Lawrence, J. Parker, J. Keeley, N. Andersen, M. VanDyken, and M. Hatfield-Eldred. 2018. Association between dementia severity and recommended lifestyle changes: A retrospective cohort study. *American Journal of Alzheimer's Disease & Other Dementias* 33(4):242–246.

Tom, S. E., R. A. Hubbard, P. K. Crane, S. J. Haneuse, J. Bowen, W. C. McCormick, S. McCurry, and E. B. Larson. 2015. Characterization of dementia and Alzheimer's disease in an older population: Updated incidence and life expectancy with and without dementia. *American Journal of Public Health* 105(2):408–413.

Tschanz, J. T., C. D. Corcoran, S. Schwartz, K. Treiber, R. C. Green, M. C. Norton, M. M. Mielke, K. Piercy, M. Steinberg, P. V. Rabins, J.-M. Leoutsakos, K. A. Welsh-Bohmer, J. C. S. Breitner, and C. G. Lyketsos. 2011. Progression of cognitive, functional, and neuropsychiatric symptom domains in a population cohort with Alzheimer dementia: The Cache County Dementia Progression study. *American Journal of Geriatric Psychiatry* 19(6):532–542.

UsAgainstAlzheimer's. 2020. *Activists against Alzheimer's.* https://www.usagainstalzheimers.org/networks/activists (accessed November 11, 2020).

Zimmerman, S., W. Anderson, S. Brode, D. Jonas, L. Lux, A. Beeber, L. Watson, M. Viswanathan, K. Lohr, J. Cook Middleton, L. Jackson, and P. Sloane. 2011. Comparison of characteristics of nursing homes and other residential long-term care settings for people with dementia. *Comparative Effectiveness Review No. 79*. Rockville, MD: Agency for Healthcare Research and Quality.

3

COMPLEXITY OF SYSTEMS FOR DEMENTIA CARE, SERVICES, AND SUPPORTS

This chapter describes the complex systems in which dementia care interventions are implemented and how these complexities factor into an assessment of the evidence derived from these interventions. It begins by describing a multilevel framework the committee used to organize the conceptualization of different kinds of care interventions for persons living with dementia and their care partners and caregivers and to aid in identifying gaps in the existing knowledge base (those gaps are discussed further in Chapter 5). The chapter then goes on to describe the challenges inherent in assessing evidence from dementia care interventions. That section ends by identifying some of the principal actors and programs that make up the complex system of dementia care in the United States.

A MULTILEVEL FRAMEWORK FOR CARE INTERVENTIONS FOR PERSONS LIVING WITH DEMENTIA AND THEIR CARE PARTNERS AND CAREGIVERS

The broad range and heterogeneity of the dementia care interventions evaluated in the Agency for Healthcare Research and Quality (AHRQ) systematic review necessitated a framework with which the committee could structure its assessment of the interventions and their readiness for broad dissemination and implementation. To this end, the committee adapted a multilevel framework previously developed to organize the literature for caregiving interventions (NASEM, 2016). The resulting framework (see Figure 3-1) depicts the multifaceted context in which dementia care is provided and received. This context encompasses a wide range of care settings

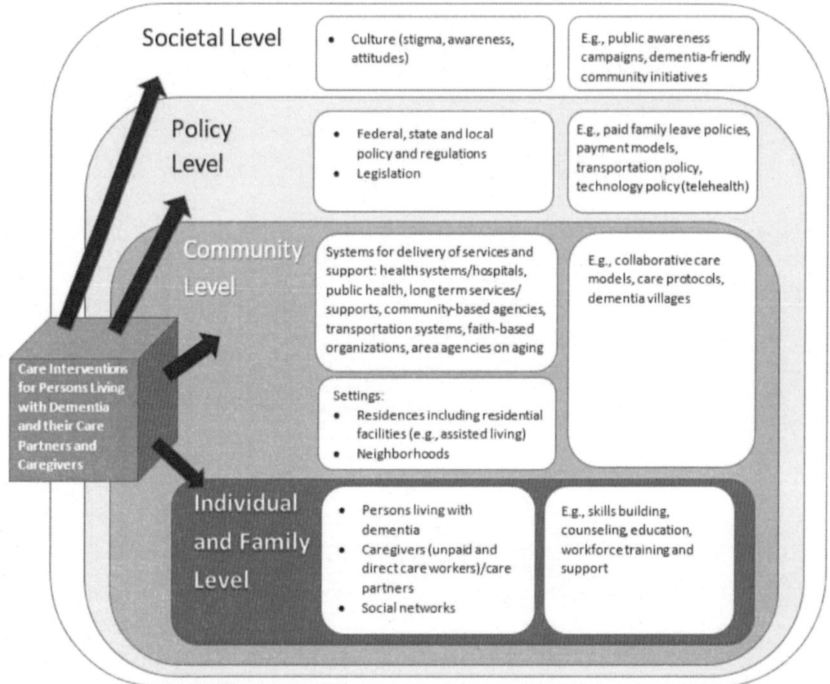

FIGURE 3-1 Organizing framework for care interventions for persons living with dementia and their care partners and caregivers.
SOURCE: Adapted from NASEM, 2016.

(e.g., private homes, residential care facilities) and significant heterogeneity in the social and community networks of persons living with dementia (e.g., family members, friends, workplaces, health care organizations, community- and faith-based organizations), as well as in the societal and policy (federal, state, and local) environments. Applying this framework allows dementia care interventions to be categorized as targeting various levels—individual and family, community, policy, and societal—either alone or in combination. As depicted in the figure, the levels are nested, and there is a dynamic interplay among them (i.e., individuals and families reside and receive care, services, and supports in communities, which in turn exist within policy environments, which are influenced by societal perceptions and cultural norms).

Individual and Family Level

Interventions at the individual and family level directly target persons living with dementia or care partners and caregivers, and are generally designed to alter some aspect of behavior or risk (e.g., depression, strain). As discussed in Chapter 2, care partners and caregivers may be family members and/or friends of the person living with dementia or paid providers. In considering interventions at this level, it is important to recognize that individual care arrangements often extend beyond a person living with dementia–caregiver dyad to a broader network of engaged family, friends, and paid caregivers. These helping networks are recognized as being dynamic in response to the evolving care needs of persons living with dementia and the circumstances of care partners and caregivers, who may be managing multiple employment and family responsibilities or may experience health or financial circumstances that affect their ability to provide care (NASEM, 2016). Many of the interventions examined in the AHRQ systematic review, such as psychosocial interventions, exercise, reminiscence therapy, and multicomponent interventions (which often include psychotherapeutic, education and skills building, and social support components), target persons living with dementia and their care partners and caregivers. Outcomes of individual- and family-level interventions examined in the existing evidence base often relate to the physical and emotional health of persons living with dementia or care partners/caregivers,[1] their knowledge and skills, the duration of care, and the economic effects on the individual or family unit. An example of an individual-level intervention is the New York University Spouse-Caregiver Intervention Study, which evaluated the effect of individual and family counseling and support (via support groups) for spouse-caregivers of persons living with Alzheimer's disease on the caregivers' depressive symptoms (Mittelman et al., 1996, 2004).

Community Level

The organizing framework depicted in Figure 3-1 conceptualizes communities broadly as encompassing a range of care and support systems, as well as residential care settings, including private homes, where persons living with dementia and their care partners and caregivers live and have the opportunity for a meaningful life. Systems in this context encompass health care, public health, social services agencies, and organizations providing long-term services and supports (LTSS).

[1] Interventions that target the health or well-being of direct care workers are categorized as individual-level interventions, but those that aim to alter process or system outcomes (e.g., training of direct care workers to improve care coordination) are addressed in the section on community-level interventions.

The committee considered systems and settings together under the broader umbrella of the community level in recognition of their matrixed nature. That is, systems that address the continuum of care, services, and supports required by persons living with dementia and their care partners and caregivers to meet functional needs and those that address public health prevention and wellness function in a multitude of care settings within communities (NQF, 2014). Some interventions at this level specifically target the interface between delivery systems and care settings. For example, dementia villages are residential settings designed and operated around the care and support needs of persons living with dementia, providing housing, food, security, opportunities for social interaction, and access to a range of medical care and LTSS (Haeusermann, 2018). Other interventions at the community level, such as collaborative care models, may be focused on altering the structure or operation of systems for delivery of services and supports. Such interventions often require adjustments to workflow or a reconfiguring of the connections between service delivery and community agencies. Relevant examples include the connections between health systems and community-based organizations (CBOs), such as an area agency on aging or a subsidized housing organization (NASEM, 2016). The framework also recognizes that communities have myriad other resources (e.g., religious and art institutions, libraries, senior centers) that can play vital roles in the support of persons living with dementia and their care partners and caregivers, although access to community institutions and the services they provide varies depending on where people live (NASEM, 2016).

Thus, interventions that target the community level are diverse and should not be considered in isolation. Note also that outcomes for community-targeted interventions may be measured at the payer (e.g., Medicare, Medicaid, private insurer), organizational (e.g., service delivery), or individual (e.g., quality of life, strain) level.

Policy Level

Interventions at the policy level include federal, state, and local legislation, regulations, and policies that affect available supports and services for persons living with dementia and their care partners and caregivers. Examples include insurance reimbursement policies, such as the structure and generosity of Medicaid coverage of LTSS; state and federal policies regarding paid and unpaid leave for caregivers (e.g., the Family and Medical Leave Act of 1993); changes to Medicare reimbursement that support dementia care planning; state and federal regulations requiring the delivery of person-centered care; and state- and federal-level dementia training requirements for certified nursing assistants and home health and home care aides (NASEM, 2016). Policy-level interventions can offer myriad benefits to persons living with dementia and their care partners and caregivers, such as reducing personal expenditures for medical care and other supports and services; increasing access to services; creating financial and quality incentives for health systems, LTSS providers, and CBOs to coordinate and integrate services; establishing expectations that the needs of caregivers of persons living with dementia will be assessed and supported; and providing employment protection for care partners and caregivers. Outcomes of such interventions may be measured at the individual, organizational, payer, or population level.

Societal Level

Societal-level interventions encompass strategies that affect how society views dementia by targeting the consciousness and perceptions of a population (e.g., awareness, stigma). Such strategies take into account the cultural variation in how dementia is defined, perceived, and addressed at the individual, community, and policy levels. For example, the stigma faced by persons living with dementia is often entangled with ageism that is pervasive in many societies (Evans, 2018). As discussed in Chapter 2, societal understanding of and views on dementia may affect policy making and decisions about investments in supports and services for persons living with dementia and their care partners and caregivers. Issues related to awareness and stigma may influence individuals' actions to seek out needed care (Hickey, 2019). Examination of societal outcomes will generally focus on population-level effects, but may encompass any geographic locality that serves as the frame for the intervention of interest. Public awareness campaigns, for example, seek to promote understanding of dementia and foster a society that is inclusive and supportive of persons living with dementia and their care partners and caregivers. Some, like Ireland's Understand Together campaign, may be focused broadly at raising awareness at the national level (Hickey, 2019), while others may aim to bring about change at the local community level (e.g., dementia-friendly communities) (Buckner et al., 2019). Persons living with dementia have played important roles in advancing societal-level interventions aimed at improving public awareness about the disease. These self-advocacy efforts, through such organizations as UsAgainstAlzheimer's, are working to promote not only improved public understanding but also support among policy makers for dementia research and care-related policies (UsAgainstAlzheimer's, 2020).

COMPLEXITY OF DEMENTIA CARE INTERVENTIONS AND IMPLICATIONS FOR ASSESSING THE EVIDENCE

The interactions and interdependencies among persons living with dementia, care partners and caregivers, the community, and the broader policy and societal environments are complex. Heterogeneity in the populations, settings, care and support systems, and policy environments in which care interventions are implemented may lead to variation in the observed effects of those interventions. Such contextual effects can obscure signals of intervention effectiveness. As discussed below, this complexity poses challenges for the assessment of evidence supporting the readiness of interventions for broad dissemination and implementation.

Health service and public health interventions, such as nonpharmacological dementia care interventions, are often described as being complex interventions (Craig et al., 2008; Minary et al., 2018). They frequently involve multiple components that are constantly interacting with each other and with the context in which the intervention is taking place. While pharmacological interventions, such as medications to control type 2 diabetes, have their own complexities (Bolen et al., 2016), the interactions between health service and public health interventions and context are especially relevant in determining the complexity of an intervention. For example, a seemingly simple exercise intervention involves not only performing exercise but also interacting socially with a trainer and learning new skills, and it may occur in varied settings (e.g., home, gym, nursing home). These inherent interactions between intervention and context make it challenging to disentangle the effects caused by the intervention from those caused by the specific context in which the intervention is occurring (Minary et al., 2018). It is important to note that the goal of disentangling intervention effects from contextual effects is not achieved by separating the intervention from its context, but by understanding how various contexts affect the outcomes of the intervention. While context effects have posed challenges to systematic evidence review methods that focus on assessing the effectiveness of an intervention, realist review methods are designed to improve understanding of the intervention mechanisms that lead to outcomes of interest and the contexts in which those mechanisms function (Pawson et al., 2005).

Complexity Related to the Heterogeneity of the Disease and Populations Affected

As is true of the general population, persons living with dementia, care partners, and caregivers exhibit heterogeneity and represent a diverse range of genders, races, ethnicities, socioeconomic backgrounds, and marital statuses. It is also important to underscore that not all causes of dementias are the same. Persons with dementia may be diagnosed with one or more dementia-causing diseases, such as Alzheimer's disease, vascular dementia, or Lewy body dementia, and the onset of related symptoms may occur earlier or later in life.

Adding to the complexity of dementia is the degenerative, dynamic, and unpredictable nature of the disease. As the symptoms of dementia progress, the needs of persons living with dementia and of their care partners and caregivers evolve, and it can be difficult to anticipate how these needs will change (Whitlatch and Orsulic-Jeras, 2018). However, studies on dementia care interventions are inconsistent in reporting of the disease stage of the target population (Butler et al., 2020), complicating understanding of how specific interventions affect persons living with dementia and their care partners and caregivers in different stages of disease progression. The broad spectrum of needs along the progression of the disease for persons living with dementia and their care partners and caregivers needs to be considered in study designs, outcomes, and reporting of results.

Measuring the outcomes of dementia care interventions is critical for having a scientific approach to designing and delivering care, services, and supports for persons living with dementia, care partners, and caregivers. Medical outcomes for persons with cancer, osteoporosis, or heart disease can be captured through such measures as fewer deaths or fractures or less breathlessness and fatigue, or via biomarkers. Persons with these conditions also frequently have quality-of-life concerns, and these outcomes are more difficult to capture. Outcomes related to quality of life and meaning are even more difficult to capture for persons living with dementia. This is due in part to the cognitive impairments they experience, particularly during the later stages of disease, and in part to the inherent goal of dementia care, services, and supports—to help a person live well in the world, which, as described above, is a personal experience that varies for persons living with dementia, care partners, and caregivers. In measuring intervention outcomes, both the person with dementia and the care partner/caregiver could be asked about this outcome, but how should these perspectives be weighed, particularly during the severe stage of disease? And what measures should be used to capture what is most important to people? Summative measures of overall well-being are attractive because they are all encompassing, but they may miss the intended target of an intervention, such as mood. In contrast, such quantifiable measures as emergency room visits may miss the mark of what matters to a person. These issues are discussed further in Chapter 6.

Complexity of Dementia Care Interventions

As discussed earlier in this chapter, some interventions may have components that span multiple levels of the framework depicted in Figure 3-1. The need for tailoring of care interventions—whether cultural tailoring or tailoring to the unique circumstances of individuals and organizations—adds another layer of complexity. As discussed further in Chapter 6, such tailoring is critical to ensuring that care interventions are accessible to and meet the needs of the full range of populations that are affected by dementia and, importantly, the individuals within those populations (Graham et al., 2006). At the same time, however, variability in implementation may also give rise to variation in outcomes.

Complexity Related to the Systems in Which Interventions Are Implemented

As noted, interventions are affected by the community, policy, and societal contexts in which they are implemented. For example, reimbursement policies can disincentivize care practitioners from spending time discussing the values, goals, and needs of persons living with dementia and their care partners and caregivers (NASEM, 2016), which may reduce the effectiveness of interventions targeting the individual level, and likely those dependent on tailoring in particular. Further complexity results from the myriad stakeholders involved in the implementation of interventions. An overview of the complex ecosystem of actors and programs that support dementia care interventions is presented in Box 3-1.

CONCLUSION

Interventions for persons living with dementia and their care partners and caregivers can be implemented at multiple levels, ranging from the individual to society. While this allows the needs of persons living with dementia and their care partners and caregivers to be addressed from various perspectives, the interactions among these levels can affect outcomes and introduce complexity into dementia care interventions. Also introducing complexity is the fact that persons living with dementia and care partners and caregivers are highly diverse, representing different ages, genders, races and ethnicities, sexual orientations and gender identities, and types and stages of dementia. Underpinning all of this complexity is that dementia care interventions are themselves often complex, involving myriad interconnected components that interact with each other and with the context and system in which they are implemented.

> CONCLUSION: *Dementia care interventions are complex as a result of the multiple levels at which they are implemented, interactions among those levels, the diversity of persons living with dementia and their care partners and caregivers, and the complexity of the interventions themselves. This complexity presents challenges to the evaluation of interventions, and limited the ability of the AHRQ systematic review to draw conclusions for many of the*

BOX 3-1
Actors and Programs for the Implementation of Evidence-Based Interventions

The ecosystem of actors and programs that support dementia care interventions is complex. An overview of some of the actors and programs is presented below.

Calls for Evidence-Based Interventions

Centers for Disease Control and Prevention

- The **Healthy Brain Initiative** supports award recipient organizations (e.g., the Alzheimer's Association) to develop and implement public health strategies based in the Healthy Brain Initiative Road Map Series, to implement and evaluate the Road Map Series, and to assist with the development of future Road Maps. Two Healthy Brain Initiative Road Maps call for the implementation of effective interventions that will help meet the needs of persons living with dementia and their care partners and caregivers:
  - **State and Local Public Health Partnerships to Address Dementia: The 2018–2023 Road Map**
  - **Road Map for Indian Country**

Office of the Assistant Secretary for Planning and Evaluation, U.S. Department of Health and Human Services

- **The 2019 Update of the National Plan to Address Alzheimer's Disease (National Plan)** outlines specific actions that include "develop and disseminate evidence-based interventions for people with Alzheimer's disease and related dementias and their caregivers," and refers to the Agency for Healthcare Research and Quality (AHRQ) systematic review and forthcoming recommendations of the present report. Another action within the National Plan is to "provide effective caregiver interventions through Alzheimer's disease and related dementias-capable systems."
- The **Advisory Council on Alzheimer's Research, Care, and Services** includes members from federal agencies as well as advocates living with dementia, care partners and caregivers, and other stakeholders. The Advisory Council meets quarterly to discuss government programs that address the needs of persons living with dementia and their care partners and caregivers, and to review and make recommendations on the priority actions within the National Plan.

Private Foundations

- Philanthropic organizations, such as The John A. Hartford Foundation and AARP Foundation, award grants to various projects that are studying the effectiveness of interventions for persons living with dementia and their care partners and caregivers.

continued

BOX 3-1 Continued

Infrastructure and Resources for Implementation and Evaluation

Administration for Community Living

- The **Alzheimer's Disease Programs Initiative** (ADPI) supports persons living with dementia and their care partners and caregivers through a combination of state- and community-level programs.
  - One of the three components of the ADPI is the forging of cooperative agreements and provision of grant funding to states and communities for the development and implementation of person-centered services and supports for persons living with dementia and their care partners and caregivers.
  - Grants are provided to home- and community-based service systems and community-based organizations that aim to translate and implement evidence-based supportive services for persons living with dementia and their care partners and caregivers at the community level.

Centers for Disease Control and Prevention (CDC)

- The Building Our Largest Dementia (BOLD) Infrastructure for Alzheimer's Act (2018) amends the Public Health Service Act, instructing CDC to establish **Alzheimer's and Related Dementias Public Health Centers of Excellence** (PHCOEs). PHCOEs translate and disseminate research through public health programs of state, local, tribal, and other partners across the country.
  - The Alzheimer's Association is the designated PHCOE for dementia risk reduction.
  - The University of Minnesota in the designated PHCOE for dementia caregiving.

U.S. Department of Veterans Affairs (VA)

- The **Program of General Caregiver Support Services** offers care partners and caregivers of persons living with dementia a variety of interventions. Care partners and caregivers of veterans or veterans who are care partners or caregivers and receive care through the VA are eligible for these interventions.

National Institute on Aging (NIA)

- Thirty-one **Alzheimer's Disease Research Centers** (ADRCs) across the United States, funded by NIA, perform translational dementia research. The ADRCs function as a network that shares research ideas, approaches, and data.
- The **IMbedded Pragmatic Alzheimer's disease and related dementias Clinical Trials (IMPACT) Collaboratory** aims to build capacity for conducting pragmatic clinical trials embedded within health care systems.

Agency for Healthcare Research and Quality (AHRQ)

- The **AHRQ Health Care Innovations Exchange** collects innovation descriptions, practical tools, and other resources to allow health professionals and researchers to share and adopt innovations in health care.
- **Practice-Based Research Networks** (PBRNs) are groups of primary care clinicians and community-based practices that collaborate to translate research results into real-world practice.

Centers for Medicare & Medicaid Services and State Medicaid Programs

- Federal and state Medicaid programs have the opportunity to expand waivers and entitlement programs for evidence-based interventions through both institutional and home- and community-based services.

Local-Level Organizations

- Local community-based organizations and networks, such as Dementia Friendly America, that work on the front lines of intervention delivery have the opportunity to expand access to evidence-based interventions by including them in their intervention offerings.

Health Care Systems

- Health care systems and networks have the opportunity to incorporate and promote evidence-based interventions within the core of routine service provision that is offered to persons living with dementia and their care partners and caregivers. Health care systems can also contribute to the continued gathering of evidence on the implementation of these interventions in diverse settings and populations.

Payment Models

Centers for Medicare & Medicaid Services (CMS)

- Through the **Innovation Center**, CMS is developing and evaluating new payment and service delivery models. As part of the Health Care Innovation Awards, four dementia care delivery models have been evaluated:
  - Care Ecosystem—The University of California, San Francisco, and the University of Nebraska Medical Center Dementia Care Ecosystem: Using Innovative Technologies to Personalize and Deliver Coordinated Dementia Care
  - Maximizing Independence at Home (MIND)—Comprehensive Home-based Dementia Care Coordination for Medicare-Medicaid Dual Eligibles in Maryland
  - The University of California, Los Angeles, Alzheimer's and Dementia Care—Comprehensive, Coordinated, Patient-Centered
  - Aging Brain Care—Dissemination of the Aging Brain Care Program
- **Special Needs Plans** are a type of Medicare Advantage Plan that provides benefits and services to individuals with certain diseases or health care needs. Special Needs Plans tailor the benefits and services offered to the

continued

BOX 3-1 Continued

groups they serve. Dementia is a qualifying condition that may enable persons living with dementia to enroll in such plans.

- The **Medicaid Innovation Accelerator Program** supports a program area in improving care for Medicaid beneficiaries with complex care needs and high costs. An arm of this program area, Beneficiaries with Complex Care Needs and High Costs (BCN) Program Support for State Medicaid Agencies, aims to facilitate the replication and spread of BCN programs.
- States that contract with Medicaid managed care organizations (MCOs) must develop a state quality strategy with input from beneficiaries and stakeholders to evaluate the care delivered through MCOs. An External Quality Review Organization then performs an External Quality Review of the contracted health plans based on each state's quality strategy.

SOURCES: AARP, 2020; ACL, 2019; AHRQ, n.d.-a, n.d.-b; Alzheimer's Association and CDC, 2018, 2019; CDC, 2020; CMS, n.d.-a, n.d.-b, n.d.-c, n.d.-d, n.d.-e, n.d.-f; Dementia Friendly America, 2018; HHS, 2019, 2020; NIA, 2020, n.d.; NIA IMPACT Collaboratory, n.d.; NORC at the University of Chicago, 2016; The John A. Hartford Foundation, 2020; VA, 2020.

interventions considered. To improve the ability to answer questions about which dementia care interventions work, for whom, and under what circumstances, future research and synthesis approaches need to account for these complexities in the design, implementation, and evaluation of interventions.

REFERENCES

AARP. 2020. *AARP community challenge 2020 grantees.* https://www.aarp.org/livable-communities/community-challenge/info-2020/2020-grantees.html (accessed November 9, 2020).

ACL (Administration for Community Living). 2019. *Support for people with dementia, including Alzheimer's disease.* https://acl.gov/programs/support-people-alzheimers-disease/support-people-dementia-including-alzheimers-disease (accessed October 13, 2020).

AHRQ (Agency for Healthcare Research and Quality). n.d.-a. *About the AHRQ health care innovations exchange.* https://innovations.ahrq.gov/about-us (accessed November 9, 2020).

AHRQ. n.d.-b. *Practice-based research networks: Research in everyday practice.* https://pbrn.ahrq.gov (accessed November 9, 2020).

Alzheimer's Association and CDC (Centers for Disease Control and Prevention). 2018. *Healthy brain initiative, state and local public health partnerships to address dementia: The 2018–2023 road map.* Chicago, IL: Alzheimer's Association.

Alzheimer's Association and CDC. 2019. *Healthy brain initiative: Road map for Indian country.* Chicago, IL: Alzheimer's Association.

Bolen, S., E. Tseng, S. Hutfless, J. Segal, C. Suarez-Cuervo, Z. Berger, L. Wilson, Y. Chu, E. Iyoha, and N. Maruthur. 2016. *Diabetes medications for adults with type 2 diabetes: An update.* Rockville, MD: Agency for Healthcare Research and Quality.

Buckner, S., N. Darlington, M. Woodward, M. Buswell, E. Mathie, A. Arthur, L. Lafortune, A. Killett, A. Mayrhofer, J. Thurman, and C. Goodman. 2019. Dementia friendly communities in England: A scoping study. *International Journal of Geriatric Psychiatry* 34(8):1235–1243.

Butler, M., J. E. Gaugler, K. M. C. Talley, H. I. Abdi, P. J. Desai, S. Duval, M. L. Forte, V. A. Nelson, W. Ng, J. M. Ouellette, E. Ratner, J. Saha, T. Shippee, B. L. Wagner, T. J. Wilt, and L. Yeshi. 2020. Care interventions for people living with dementia and their caregivers. *Comparative Effectiveness Review No. 231.* Rockville, MD: Agency for Healthcare Research and Quality. doi: 10.23970/AHRQEPCCER231.

CDC (Centers for Disease Control and Prevention). 2020. *BOLD public health centers of excellence recipients.* https://www.cdc.gov/aging/funding/phc/index.html (accessed October 13, 2020).

CMS (Centers for Medicare & Medicaid Services). n.d.-a. *Home & community-based services 1915(c).* https://www.medicaid.gov/medicaid/home-community-based-services/home-community-based-services-authorities/home-community-based-services-1915c/index.html (accessed October 22, 2020).

CMS. n.d.-b. *Improving care for Medicaid beneficiaries with complex care needs and high costs.* https://www.medicaid.gov/resources-for-states/innovation-accelerator-program/program-areas/improving-care-for-medicaid-beneficiaries-complex-care-needs-and-high-costs/index.html (accessed October 13, 2020).

CMS. n.d.-c. *Innovation models.* https://innovation.cms.gov/innovation-models#views=models (accessed October 13, 2020).

CMS. n.d.-d. *Institutional long term care.* https://www.medicaid.gov/medicaid/long-term-services-supports/institutional-long-term-care/index.html (accessed October 22, 2020).

CMS. n.d.-e. *Quality of care external quality review.* https://www.medicaid.gov/medicaid/quality-of-care/medicaid-managed-care/quality-of-care-external-quality-review/index.html (accessed October 13, 2020).

CMS. n.d.-f. *Special needs plans (SNP).* https://www.medicare.gov/sign-up-change-plans/types-of-medicare-health-plans/special-needs-plans-snp (accessed October 13, 2020).

Craig, P., P. Dieppe, S. Macintyre, S. Michie, I. Nazareth, and M. Petticrew. 2008. Developing and evaluating complex interventions: The new medical research council guidance. *BMJ* 337:a1655.

Dementia Friendly America. 2018. *About dementia friendly America.* https://www.dfamerica.org/what-is-dfa (accessed October 21, 2020).

Evans, S. C. 2018. Ageism and dementia. In *Contemporary perspectives on ageism*, edited by L. Ayalon and C. Tesch-Römer. Cham, Switzerland: Springer International Publishing. Pp. 263–275.

Graham, I. D., J. Logan, M. B. Harrison, S. E. Straus, J. Tetroe, W. Caswell, and N. Robinson. 2006. Lost in knowledge translation: Time for a map? *Journal of Continuing Education in the Health Professions* 26(1):13–24.

Haeusermann, T. 2018. The dementia village: Between community and society. In *Care in healthcare: Reflections on theory and practice*, edited by F. Krause and J. Boldt. Cham: Palgrave Macmillan. Pp. 135–167.

HHS (U.S. Department of Health and Human Services). 2019. *National plan to address Alzheimer's disease: 2019 update.* https://aspe.hhs.gov/system/files/pdf/262601/NatlPlan2019.pdf (accessed October 1, 2020).

HHS. 2020. *Advisory council on Alzheimer's research, care, and services*. https://aspe.hhs.gov/advisory-council-alzheimers-research-care-and-services#:~:text=The%20Advisory%20Council%20consists%20of,dementias%20(AD%2FADRD) (accessed October 13, 2020).

Hickey, D. 2019. The impact of a national public awareness campaign on dementia knowledge and help-seeking intention in Ireland. *European Journal of Public Health* 29(4):234.

Minary, L., F. Alla, L. Cambon, J. Kivits, and L. Potvin. 2018. Addressing complexity in population health intervention research: The context/intervention interface. *Journal of Epidemiology and Community Health* 72(4):319.

Mittelman, M. S., S. H. Ferris, E. Shulman, G. Steinberg, and B. Levin. 1996. A family intervention to delay nursing home placement of patients with Alzheimer disease: A randomized controlled trial. *Journal of the American Medical Association* 276(21):1725–1731.

Mittelman, M. S., D. L. Roth, D. W. Coon, and W. E. Haley. 2004. Sustained benefit of supportive intervention for depressive symptoms in caregivers of patients with Alzheimer's disease. *American Journal of Psychiatry* 161(5):850–856.

NASEM (National Academies of Sciences, Engineering, and Medicine). 2016. *Families caring for an aging America*. Washington, DC: The National Academies Press.

NIA (National Institute on Aging). 2020. *Summit virtual meeting series: 2020 National Research Summit on Care, Services, and Supports for Persons with Dementia and Their Caregivers*. https://www.nia.nih.gov/2020-dementia-care-summit#Registration (accessed September 1, 2020).

NIA. n.d. *Alzheimer's disease research centers*. https://www.nia.nih.gov/research/adc (accessed October 13, 2020).

NIA IMPACT Collaboratory. n.d. *Overview*. https://impactcollaboratory.org/overview (accessed September 1, 2020).

NORC at the University of Chicago. 2016. *Third annual report: HCIA disease-specific evaluation*. Bethesda, MD: NORC at the University of Chicago.

NQF (National Quality Forum). 2014. *Priority setting for healthcare performance measurement: Addressing performance measure gaps for dementia, including Alzheimer's disease*. http://www.qualityforum.org/priority_setting_for_healthcare_performance_measurement_alzheimers_disease.aspx (accessed September 4, 2020).

Pawson, R., T. Greenhalgh, G. Harvey, and K. Walshe. 2005. Realist review—A new method of systematic review designed for complex policy interventions. *Journal of Health Services Research & Policy* 10(Suppl 1):21–34.

The John A. Hartford Foundation. 2020. *Recent grants*. https://www.johnahartford.org/grants-strategy (accessed November 9, 2020).

UsAgainstAlzheimer's. 2020. *Activists against Alzheimer's*. https://www.usagainstalzheimers.org/networks/activists (accessed November 11, 2020).

VA (U.S. Department of Veterans Affairs). 2020. *Program of general caregiver support services (PGCSS)*. https://www.caregiver.va.gov/Care_Caregivers.asp (accessed September 29, 2020).

Whitlatch, C. J., and S. Orsulic-Jeras. 2018. Meeting the informational, educational, and psychosocial support needs of persons living with dementia and their family caregivers. *Gerontologist* 58(Suppl 1):S58–S73.

4

MAKING DECISIONS ABOUT IMPLEMENTATION

Given the broad array of care interventions, services, and supports that have been developed for persons living with dementia and their care partners and caregivers and the varying degree to which these interventions are supported by evidence of efficacy, stakeholders in dementia care face challenging decisions regarding whether and how to implement a given intervention. How these decisions are made, including the type of evidence and other information taken into account, will vary for different stakeholders, such as persons living with dementia, care partners and caregivers, health care and long-term services and supports (LTSS) providers, care systems, payers, and policy makers. Innovative, evidence-based models of dementia care often are not widely deployed or put to broad practical use in care settings (Gitlin et al., 2015), and those interventions that are implemented often lack a strong evidence base supporting their use (Lourida et al., 2017). Many providers and consumers, moreover, have little information about the interventions available to them.

Different processes are used to develop the evidence base for nonpharmacological and pharmaceutical interventions for dementia care. Once efficacy has been established for a nonpharmacological intervention, implementation testing in real-world care settings is required to define the benefit of the intervention in actual care settings in preparation for its widespread dissemination. Implementation testing builds the evidence base on just what benefits the intervention provides under which conditions. It also helps identify adaptations that may be needed for the intervention's successful application within different systems of care, organizational structures, workflows, payment models, and cultures, and can assist decision makers in anticipating the resources required to implement and sustain the intervention in their own care systems (Sohn et al., 2020). The sustainability of an intervention being implemented in a facility, organization, or system is an important consideration, as the dynamic nature of dementia care practice requires the allocation of limited resources to proven interventions and an understanding of the integration of interventions into particular systems and organizations (Walugembe et al., 2019). Studying approaches for dissemination is also an important component of implementation testing.

In considering which dementia care interventions, services, and supports are ready for dissemination and implementation on a broad scale, the committee sought to understand the implementation science behind the translation of evidence-based interventions into routine practice in care settings, as well as in the community (i.e., by persons living with dementia and their care partners and caregivers). Reviews of the salient literature reveal few published reports on the implementation of evidence-based dementia care interventions (Gitlin et al., 2015; Lourida et al., 2017), despite evidence that both individual and contextual factors can alter the effectiveness of an intervention in achieving desired outcomes (Unützer et al., 2020). Accordingly, the committee's deliberations on implementation issues were further informed by discussions with experts in implementation science and with representatives of care systems, payers, and advocacy organizations and associations that took place during the public workshop held for this study (see Appendix B).

APPLYING IMPLEMENTATION SCIENCE[1]

Implementation science is the study of methods and strategies for promoting the translation of research findings and evidence-based practices and interventions into routine care and policy (Eccles and Mittman, 2006; University of Washington, 2020). Research in implementation science strives to understand what facilitates adoption of an intervention by end users, as well as what creates barriers to its uptake. Applying implementation science to the growing body of interventions for dementia care reveals that stakeholders consider many types of information in addition to effectiveness when making decisions about whether and how to implement these interventions in the real world. Care and service providers, as well as payers, also may consider such metrics as costs, return on investment, value, and quality indicators (Lees Haggerty et al., 2020; Teisberg et al., 2020).

[1] Some of the content of this section was drawn from the committee's discussion with two experts in implementation science research—Laura Gitlin of Drexel University and Melissa Simon of Northwestern University—which took place during the public workshop held on April 15, 2020. See Appendix B for the public workshop agenda.

Ultimately, it is the organization implementing or individuals receiving an intervention—not the intervention's developer—that determine its value or "relative advantage" (Rogers, 2003) (see Figure 4-1). That value derives from the benefits or outcomes that end users perceive they are receiving from use of the intervention. An intervention might be chosen, for example, because, compared with other interventions, it saves time, is convenient or hassle-free, offers greater patient satisfaction, or has a good reputation or image (Callahan et al., 2018). It is therefore important to identify those stakeholders and end users (e.g., persons living with dementia, care partners and caregivers, health care and LTSS providers, care systems, payers, policy makers) who hold the decision-making power and to understand what qualities they value in an intervention (Callahan et al., 2018; Gitlin et al., 2015).

Frameworks for Implementing and Evaluating Interventions in Complex Systems

The paucity of published reports describing the translation of research on dementia care interventions into practice hinders the advancement of translation efforts (Gitlin et al., 2015). Reviews of dementia care intervention studies that report on implementation efforts have found that a theory or framework is often used to facilitate practice change and audit translation success. This section describes a few of the many theoretical frameworks available for evaluating translation efforts and understanding the facilitators of and barriers to implementation (Gitlin et al., 2015).

One instrument commonly used to evaluate translation in implementation science and health services research is the Reach, Effectiveness, Adoption, Implementation, and Maintenance (RE-AIM) framework, designed to facilitate the translation of scientific evidence into public health impact and policy by increasing transparency in research and reevaluating the balance between internal validity and external validity (generalizability) (Glasgow et al., 2019). RE-AIM has been used in several studies evaluating dementia interventions (Gitlin et al., 2015; Lourida et al., 2017).

Another framework used in the field of implementation science is Normalization Process Theory (NPT), which lays out specific factors researchers might consider when incorporating and evaluating complex interventions in practice, posing questions related to coherence, cognitive participation or engagement, collective action, and reflexive monitoring (Murray et al., 2010). This framework, which considers the interactions of individual- and organizational-level factors, helps identify factors within these four components that enable or inhibit the normalization of complex interventions or their full integration into routine practice. NPT argues for considering how interventions can be sustained in practice from the start of their development.

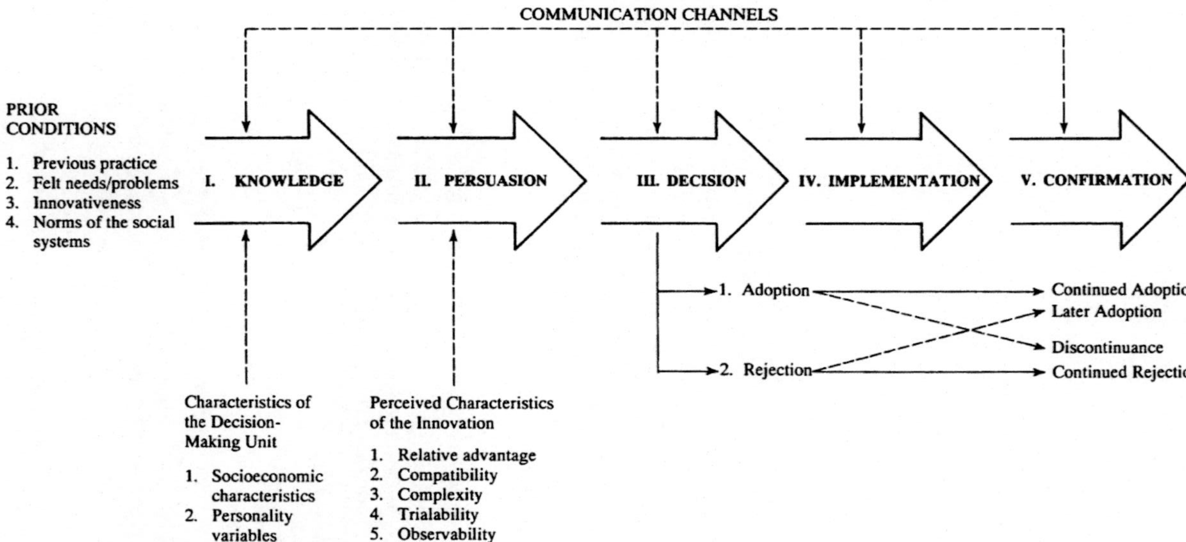

FIGURE 4-1 Rogers's model of the diffusion of innovations.
SOURCE: DIFFUSION OF INNOVATIONS, 5E by Everett M. Rogers.

Other frameworks take into account the complexities of health care delivery, potential barriers to implementation, and stakeholder perspectives on value. One example is the Agile Implementation Framework, developed by Indiana University. This framework reprioritizes eight implementation steps, so that the process starts with proactive assessment of the demand from end users rather than with the innovator's perspective and then directs the development of a scalable, sustainable solution accordingly. The framework facilitates tailoring of an intervention to the local environment; timely feedback and process modification; monitoring and assessment of impact, unintended consequences, and emergent behaviors that promote or deter uptake; and regularly updated documentation of the process to facilitate the spread and scaling of the intervention (Boustani et al., 2018; Callahan et al., 2018). This framework has been demonstrated in the implementation of a sustained collaborative dementia care model (Boustani et al., 2018).

Curran and colleagues (2012) propose a hybrid approach to study design that combines components of clinical effectiveness and implementation research to allow for more rapid translational gains, effective implementation strategies, and useful information for decision makers. They describe three hybrid models: (1) test a clinical intervention while collecting information on its delivery and implementation, (2) simultaneously test both a clinical intervention and an implementation intervention or strategy, and (3) test an implementation intervention or strategy while collecting information on the clinical intervention and its outcomes (Curran et al., 2012).

Proctor and colleagues (2011) developed a taxonomy of eight implementation outcomes—acceptability, adoption, appropriateness, feasibility, fidelity, implementation cost, penetration, and sustainability. Researchers can use this taxonomy to conceptualize and evaluate the implementation of an intervention (Proctor et al., 2011).

Carroll and colleagues (2007) provide a conceptual framework for implementation fidelity. They describe three areas of evaluation: (1) adherence (content, coverage, frequency, and duration); (2) moderators that might influence fidelity (intervention complexity, facilitation strategies, quality of delivery, and participant responsiveness); and (3) identification of essential components (i.e., components of the intervention that have the most impact) (Carroll et al., 2007).

Finally, the Consolidated Framework for Implementation Research (CFIR), developed by Damschroder and colleagues (2009), synthesizes existing theoretical frameworks to produce a list of constructs that guide researchers to examine what works, where, and why across multiple contexts. The 37 CFIR constructs fall within five major domains: intervention characteristics, outer setting, inner setting, characteristics of the individuals involved, and the implementation process (Damschroder et al., 2009).

Barriers to Implementation

Many of the barriers to the uptake of new models of dementia care, services, and supports that have been described are organizational, often revolving around workforce issues and workload/time constraints (Lourida et al., 2017). Implementing a new model might require redesigning practice, redefining professional roles, providing training for existing staff, or hiring new personnel. The ability to integrate a new care model into practice and to train or hire the necessary workforce is also impacted by the model's complexity. In some cases, a shortage of qualified personnel (e.g., limited availability of behavioral health professionals with expertise in dementia) presents a barrier. Higher rates of staff turnover have also been described as a barrier to implementation, decreasing fidelity to an intervention's defined practice model (Woltmann et al., 2008). Costs and financial sustainability can be additional considerations in deciding to implement a new model of care. There may be start-up costs (e.g., the need to acquire technology or adapt infrastructure), or coverage by third-party payers may be insufficient (Callahan et al., 2018; Lees Haggerty et al., 2020). Moreover, the pace of uptake of new models of care is impacted by the extent to which implementation requires changes in organizational culture or coordination across departments (Bradley et al., 2004; Proctor et al., 2011).

Challenges persist for those implementing evidence-based interventions that could improve the quality of life for both persons living with dementia and their care partners and caregivers. Many persons living with dementia, care partners and caregivers, and providers are not aware of or able to access these interventions. Another challenge is the clinical relevance of the evidence. For example, interventions being studied for dementia care are often not classified according to disease stage or etiology, making it difficult for providers to identify interventions that might achieve a desired outcome for a given patient at a particular stage of disease (Gitlin et al., 2015). Information on the use of interventions in demographic subgroups is also limited.

Still another challenge is that studies often do not discuss the clinical significance of the findings they are reporting—that is, whether the effect being demonstrated really matters to stakeholders. There is often little information available about the cost of implementing an intervention or about its cost-effectiveness, potential cost savings, or what burden of cost families are willing to bear to realize desired outcomes. Furthermore, not all studies consider outcomes that might be considered meaningful by caregivers, such as outcomes that improve their quality of life and reduce the personal, physical, and financial burdens of caring for a person living with dementia, or address other unmet care needs (Gitlin et al., 2015).

Underlying many of the barriers to implementation are core differences in priorities. The research process prioritizes the discovery of new and, ideally, generalizable knowledge, and is not necessarily focused on pragmatic application in real-world settings. Furthermore, few scientists in the field of aging research have expertise in implementation science. A challenge in the field of dementia care research is bridging researchers' expectation that the implementation and dissemination of their interventions will be taken up by other parties, which is often not the case (Callahan et al., 2018), and the demand for effective interventions. Policy makers, practitioners, persons living with dementia, and care partners and caregivers prioritize knowledge about practical ways to apply interventions in their context. Although the purpose of developing dementia care interventions is to meet the needs of persons living with dementia, care partners, and caregivers, they are rarely consulted or engaged in the development or implementation process. This represents a lost opportunity for researchers to allow persons living with dementia, care partners, and caregivers to determine the outcomes that matter to them and should be measured. This lack of up-front consideration of dissemination and implementation during intervention design is a key barrier that some intervention development models are working to address. The National Institute on Aging's (NIA's) IMbedded Pragmatic Alzheimer's disease and Alzheimer's disease–related dementias Clinical Trials (IMPACT) Collaboratory has begun to address this barrier by promoting embedded pragmatic clinical trials to evaluate dementia care interventions in real-world health care systems. Nonetheless, much work remains to be done to bridge the gap in priorities between health services researchers and the individuals who want access to effective interventions.

Facilitators of Implementation

The National Institutes of Health (NIH) Stage Model for Behavioral Intervention Development is a six-stage process designed to facilitate the production of "highly potent and maximally implementable behavioral interventions that improve health and well-being" (NIA, 2018). The six stages of the model are

- Stage 0: basic science research that occurs prior to intervention development;
- Stage I: activities related to the creation and preliminary testing of an intervention;
- Stage II: pure efficacy research that involves experimental testing of interventions in research settings with research-based providers;
- Stage III: real-world efficacy research that involves experimental testing in community settings with community-based providers, while still maintaining control to establish internal validity;

- Stage IV: effectiveness research in community settings with community-based providers that aims to maximize external validity; and
- Stage V: implementation and dissemination research that examines strategies of adopting an intervention in community settings.

According to the model, "intervention development is not complete until an intervention reaches its maximum level of potency *and* is implementable with a maximum number of individuals in the population for which it was developed," and the model specifically calls for implementation to be considered in the early stages of development (NIA, 2018).

Conditions that have been identified as being supportive of the uptake and implementation of new care models by organizations include alignment with health system priorities, buy-in and managerial support by organizational leadership, clinical leaders who champion the model, workforce education and training, sustainable funding/financial resources, and a dedicated infrastructure for translation activities (Bradley et al., 2004; Callahan et al., 2018; Lourida et al., 2017). The NIH Stage Model emphasizes that designing training and supervisory materials is an essential part of intervention development, helping to ensure that an intervention is administered with fidelity by providers or caregivers (NIA, 2018). There are also external factors, such as regulatory compliance, reimbursement incentives, and market pressures, that can compel implementation (Bradley et al., 2004).

The evolution of the health care payment system from a fee-for-service to a value-based model has been described as a positive development for the implementation of evidence-based dementia care. The Population Health Value framework was designed to create value and reduce costs by developing targeted pathways to care for patient populations with high expenses due to chronic conditions, including individuals living with dementia (Gupta et al., 2019). Yet, the current reimbursement system for dementia care has numerous gaps and does not cover the delivery of many of the evidence-based care models that a care plan might include. Notably, Medicare offers very limited reimbursement for LTSS (Colello, 2018). New payment models specific to dementia care have therefore been proposed. In 2017, for example, the Centers for Medicare & Medicaid Services (CMS) added a new reimbursement benefit covering the development of a written care plan for individuals with Alzheimer's disease and other dementias and cognitive disorders (Borson et al., 2017). This benefit provides for assessment and care planning, but its scope is limited, excluding ongoing care management services. In fact, services are covered only if they are provided by selected medical professionals, and not if they are provided by community-based organizations or in the context of collaborative dementia care models. One proposal to close this gap is an alternative payment model covering care management services for community-dwelling persons living with dementia.

This model would provide a per-beneficiary, per-month payment to beneficiaries, and would also provide services, education, and support to their unpaid caregivers (Boustani et al., 2019).

Finally, as noted earlier, involving all relevant stakeholders early on in the development of dementia care interventions has been discussed as an approach to reducing the barriers to dissemination and implementation (Callahan et al., 2018; Gitlin et al., 2015). By partnering with stakeholders up front, researchers can better understand the context of use of an intervention and the potential end users' needs and decision-making processes (i.e., the demand).

Deciding Whether and How to Implement an Intervention

The care delivery system has been described as a complex adaptive system in which networks of stakeholders coevolve within a changing environment. Implementing new interventions and evaluating their performance in both complex health care and public health systems is challenging, and traditional randomized controlled trials or systematic reviews are often not well suited to the task (Boustani et al., 2010; Rutter et al., 2017). There is no consensus around what constitutes sufficient evidence for deciding which interventions should advance to the implementation testing stage and dissemination. Furthermore, different studies use different methodologies to assess the evidence, and methods for evaluating the extent to which a methodology or metric is relevant to dementia care do not currently exist.

Tools have been developed to aid clinicians, policy makers, and other stakeholders in rating the quality of the available evidence as they make and implement recommendations and decisions that will guide care. One widely used decision tool is the Grading of Recommendations Assessment, Development and Evaluation (GRADE) group's Evidence to Decision (EtD) framework which can be applied to making and using clinical recommendations, coverage decisions, and health system and public health recommendations and decisions (Alonso-Coello et al., 2016; Moberg et al., 2018). This framework takes systematic reviewers and decision makers through a structured and transparent process of formulating a question based on a defined problem, making an evidence-based assessment, and drawing conclusions based on the best available research evidence. Factors taken into account in the assessment go beyond effectiveness and can include the priority of the problem, how substantial the benefits and harms of the intervention or option in question are, the certainty of the evidence, the value of the outcomes to stakeholders, how the intervention or option compares with others, resource requirements, cost-effectiveness versus comparable options, the impact on health equity, the acceptability of the intervention or option to stakeholders, and the feasibility of implementation. Conclusions drawn from the assessment might also include guidance for implementation and recommendations for monitoring and evaluation (Moberg et al., 2018). It is essential for care decisions to be based on the available evidence, and frameworks such as GRADE EtD not only support the experts who make those decisions but also help those affected by the decision understand why and how a decision was made (i.e., the strength of the evidence on which it was based) as they work to implement it in their specific circumstances. The GRADE EtD framework is discussed in greater detail and applied to specific interventions in Chapter 5.

There is also an evolving approach to systematic review in support of decision making on health interventions that incorporates a complex interventions and systems-oriented perspective (Petticrew et al., 2019). This perspective may be particularly useful when an intervention consists of multiple components, when the casual pathway between intervention and outcome is not linear, or when the effects of the intervention are context-dependent.

Monitoring and Evaluation, Quality Improvement, and Information Sharing

Given that much of the learning and knowledge generation for complex systems occurs in local and individual settings, monitoring and evaluation are crucial components of intervention implementation that need to be considered from the outset of intervention development (NAE, 2011). Monitoring can be considered an ongoing activity carried out throughout the implementation process to track the performance of an intervention by measuring inputs, such as financial and staff resources, and outputs, such as services provided and the intervention's coverage (WHO, 2004). Monitoring is often performed by the staff who are implementing the intervention. Evaluation is an episodic assessment that can be performed by project staff, sponsors, or an external third party, aimed at understanding the intervention's effect in producing specified outcomes (WHO, 2004). The outcomes targeted by these evaluations can be categorized broadly as (1) process outcomes (e.g., the intervention's content, coverage, or quality); (2) short-term outcomes (e.g., behavior, depression, cost-effectiveness); or (3) long-term impact (e.g., quality of life). It is important that monitoring and evaluation encompass both anticipated benefits of the targeted outcome and any unintended consequences that worsen the care of a condition or a system outside of the targeted area.

A preimplementation assessment of the capacities and needs of the individuals and organizations involved in the intervention can help identify barriers to and facilitators of implementation, as well as areas that may require closer monitoring during implementation (Damschroder et al., 2009). Similarly, the monitoring of progress during implementation and the collection of real-time data are important to detect unanticipated barriers to or facilitators of implementation, as well as to identify and address any potential problems before they can compromise the intervention's viability. The data collected may include both quantitative and qualitative information gathered through reflection, debriefs, and feedback among intervention staff regarding the progress and quality of implementation, discussions that can also promote shared learning and quality improvement as the implementation proceeds. In addition to ongoing monitoring, evaluations of clinical outcomes and formative evaluations are critical to understand the processes by which the intervention is implemented, the financial resources required, how context modifies effectiveness, and how the intervention can be optimized for other contexts (Curran et al., 2012; Damschroder et al., 2009; Proctor et al., 2011). It is essential for formative evaluations to be designed to assess the perceptions of stakeholders delivering and receiving the intervention, such as persons living with dementia, care partners and caregivers, providers, and administrators (Curran et al., 2012; Damschroder et al., 2009). In some instances, evaluations may be informative in indicating that there is little chance of successful implementation, and resources could better be used elsewhere (Murray et al., 2010).

To support monitoring, evaluation, and quality improvement, data will ideally be gathered from clinical research as well as clinical encounters and other services and supports settings in the community. These data will then be stored and shared among various settings involved in the delivery of care, services, and supports to persons living with dementia, care partners, and caregivers (IOM, 2013). To improve the data collection, implementers can leverage health information technology—for example, using information that is already collected in electronic health records. Patient-generated health data, provided directly by intervention participants or their designees, are another rich source of information about patients' health-related experiences and concerns in daily life (IOM, 2015).

To support comprehensive understanding of an intervention's implementation, it is important to collect performance and quality data across the spectrum of care settings, including medical care and LTSS (NASEM, 2016). The National Strategy for Quality Improvement, developed by the U.S. Department of Health and Human Services (HHS), advocates for transparent, accountable, person-centered, and higher-quality care through partnerships between provider networks and across varying settings. According to a previous report of the National Academies, however, these attributes often are not present in quality measurement practices. Within HHS, CMS, the Agency for Healthcare Research and Quality (AHRQ), and the Centers for Disease Control and Prevention (CDC) are some of the federal agencies working specifically on health data quality improvement efforts (IOM, 2015). The National Quality Forum has also recommended priorities for addressing gaps in the quality assessment of home- and community-based services, including the integration of quality data with encounter, authorization, and administrative data to facilitate the use of real-time data collection to support quality improvement (NQF, 2016). Importantly, long-term care facilities and community-based providers, which operate outside of traditional health systems that routinely collect clinical and personal data, need a data infrastructure capable of capturing and sharing data that can be used to improve the quality of care (IOM, 2015). An Electronic Long-Term Services and Supports Plan that was part of CMS's Testing Experience and Functional Tools demonstration showed promise for harmonization of data and coordination across care settings (The Lewin Group, 2018).

UNDERSTANDING DEMAND: STAKEHOLDER PERSPECTIVES ON DECISION MAKING[2]

During its public information-gathering workshop, the committee heard on-the-ground perspectives from stakeholders in dementia care, including representatives of advocacy organizations and associations and care systems and payers.

Advocacy Organizations and Associations

Representatives of advocacy organizations and associations expressed to the committee their view that persons living with dementia and their care partners and caregivers need interventions and support now. They stated that decisions regarding which interventions to try, for which individuals, in which situations, with the available resources are being made using the best evidence currently available. Ideally, the selection of interventions would be based on rigorous evidence of effectiveness, but lacking that evidence, decision makers take a range of individual, interventional, and contextual criteria and characteristics into consideration.

Lynn Feinberg of AARP shared her perspective that the main barriers to scaling up evidence-based dementia interventions are the lack of technical assistance and guidelines for providers in determining which caregivers could benefit from which interventions; the lack of up-front consideration of dissemination and implementation during intervention design; and the

[2] The content of this section was drawn from the committee's discussions with representatives of advocacy organizations and associations and care systems and payers that took place during the public workshop held on April 15, 2020. See Appendix B for the public workshop agenda.

lack of sufficient funding and payment mechanisms covering evidence-based caregiver support services in practice settings. Despite the persistent gaps in the implementation evidence base for dementia care interventions, persons living with dementia and care partners and caregivers must move forward and make *evidence-informed* decisions regarding the available interventions. The view Feinberg expressed to the committee is that the need for more rigorous research should not delay the scale-up and promotion of evidence-informed practices and caregiver support services and programs for families that need help.

Kathleen Kelly of Family Caregiver Alliance stated that care situations are dynamic, and the Alliance looks to identify interventions and supports that meet a dementia caregiver's needs wherever they fall along the spectrum of care. The Alliance conducts a uniform assessment to develop a care plan tailored to the needs of the family, and moves forward using the best evidence-based interventions available at the time. Unfortunately, where an intervention fits best along the spectrum of care is not always clear, and efforts are further hampered by the lack of a common language for assessment of caregiver needs. Practical issues of intervention implementation also need to be considered, such as staffing needs (e.g., whether the intervention is delivered in a group or one-to-one); training needs (and whether a training or operations manual or technical assistance is available); and resource needs (e.g., whether app, online, or telehealth resources are available and whether the family has access to the Internet).

Douglas Pace of the Alzheimer's Association highlighted the finding from the AHRQ systematic review that insufficient evidence of an intervention's effectiveness does not equate to its being ineffective. He emphasized the importance of ensuring that interventions remain available to those who find them helpful while the evidence base to support more widespread dissemination is being assembled. He pointed out that many care interventions are ready for dissemination, and for others, existing data can be leveraged and shared collaboratively to grow the evidence base. In considering which interventions to try, it is important to consider the desires of persons living with dementia and care partners and caregivers and the accessibility of the interventions to them. For example, "short-term low-touch interventions" are needed in conjunction with or as an alternative to more comprehensive programs and services.

In reflecting on the five domains in which the AHRQ review assessed the strength of the evidence base for interventions (study limitations, consistency, directness, precision, reporting bias), Kelly, Pace, and Feinberg each indicated that criteria related to consistency and directness (a direct link between intervention and outcome) were the most important contributors to their organization's decision-making process. The recommendations of the Service Providers Stakeholder Group at the 2020 Research Summit on Dementia Care were also noted,[3] and Pace emphasized the underlying recommendation themes of person-centered care and diversity, equity, and inclusion in the development, evaluation, dissemination, and implementation of dementia care interventions.

Care Systems and Payers

Representatives of care systems and payers expressed opinions similar to those of other stakeholders regarding elements of decision making.[4] Payers are particularly interested in whether interventions are consistently achieving the intended outcomes in the intended population, as integrated in the care system and implemented by the end user.

Patrick Courneya of HealthPartners suggested that implementation and dissemination decisions sit at the intersection of what is determined to be of value based on evidence of efficacy and what is meaningful to individuals and their personal experiences and circumstances. The principle of "first do no harm" must be balanced against the strength of the evidence for whether an intervention does or does not work. According to Courneya, there is an opportunity to create infrastructure for the collection of pragmatic, real-world information about the effectiveness of organizations and service providers in delivering covered services consistently, and about whether the intervention's delivery is having the intended impact in the community or there are any unanticipated effects. From a decision-making perspective, it is important to understand who specifically derives benefits from the intervention (e.g., persons living with dementia, care partners and caregivers, employers, society, other stakeholders). Payers take into account how widely available the intervention is, the associated costs, and how it compares with other approaches. Other considerations might include how practicable and logistically feasible an intervention is, whether it can be deployed with fidelity, and whether its performance can be reliably monitored.

David Gifford of the American Health Care Association said he often hears from providers that interventions supported by a solid evidence base are not effective in their hands. He attributed this disconnect not to issues with the evidence but to problems with workflow, integration, and implementation. To be successful, tools and strategies must be integrated within the health care delivery system, and this aspect of an intervention

[3] More information about the summit and recommendations developed by the Service Providers Stakeholder Group is available at https://aspe.hhs.gov/research-summit-dementia-care-2020-stakeholder-groups (accessed August 18, 2020).

[4] More information about the summit and recommendations developed by the Payer Stakeholder Group is available at https://aspe.hhs.gov/research-summit-dementia-care-2020-stakeholder groups (accessed August 18, 2020).

is often overlooked. Another consideration for implementation is the type of intervention. Pharmaceutical products that target the pathophysiology of dementia are not necessarily the type of intervention that will provide the desired outcome for an individual grappling with a lost function or cognitive domain. With regard to decision making, providers and policy makers bypass studies that conclude only that more study is needed, and they gravitate toward those studies that do draw a conclusion, even if the evidence is poor. According to Gifford, the evidence base used by decision makers would benefit from researchers drawing conclusions when possible, with caveats if needed.

Lewis Sandy of UnitedHealth Group pointed out that many persons living with dementia are Medicare beneficiaries, as are many care partners and caregivers. Thus, when considering who will be implementing dementia care interventions, it is important to understand how Medicare operates. Whereas what can be covered by traditional Medicare is governed by statute and regulation, Medicare Advantage plans have more flexibility to offer additional benefits, and many provide in-home support, telemonitoring, and support for caregivers. There are special needs plans for those with chronic health conditions; however, very few of these plans are targeted toward dementia. From a payer perspective, evidence that might not meet the evidentiary standards for publication or is not statistically significant can still be of interest to inform their decisions. Payers are particularly interested in interventions that are ready to scale and have been demonstrated to be robust across a range of implementation conditions (e.g., populations, geographies, care settings).

Shari Ling of CMS said that a challenge for CMS is making decisions based on an evidence base that varies widely in the outcomes reported. The Medicare population lives with multiple comorbidities, and it would be helpful to have a core set of meaningful outcome measures to help align the science with practice and policy. It would also be helpful to define universal processes and indices of outcomes that are meaningful for caregivers and could be incorporated into clinical trials. When considering readiness for implementation, it is important to identify who will implement an intervention (e.g., persons living with dementia, care partners/caregivers, clinicians, practices, systems) and understand how they will use it (including how it will fit into the workflow). Medicare is defined by statute, and CMS must adhere to program and policy implementation levers when deploying interventions. When deciding about coverage, for example, CMS must look for evidence that an intervention meaningfully improves outcomes in the intended population. In this case, it is important for the target population to be clearly defined. Quality measurement requires having a clearly defined numerator (the outcome to be achieved) and denominator (the population in which it is to be achieved). In the work of the CMS Innovation Center, it must be demonstrated that care models and payment models are achieving improved quality.

Workshop participants also discussed the level of evidence needed and other considerations in deciding whether to launch an embedded pragmatic clinical trial, noting that buy-in from providers and organizational leadership is essential for trial success. Considerations include the burden the trial will impose on providers who will have to implement the intervention for the trial (e.g., whether the intervention will integrate into the existing workflow); the potential scalability of the intervention; and the adaptability of the trial design, as adaptable designs are more likely to yield useful results. Cost considerations for both care systems and payers include not only the costs of the intervention itself but also the costs entailed at every step in the implementation process, from identifying and then engaging the target population for the intervention, to delivering the intervention with fidelity, to carrying out measurement and evaluation. Cost savings that an intervention may offer to payers or providers are also a consideration (and are a mandated consideration for programs of the CMS Innovation Center).

CONCLUSIONS

Given the complexity of dementia care interventions, it is challenging to evaluate how and under what circumstances they can be implemented to move the evidence base beyond efficacy and even pragmatic trials toward readiness for implementation and dissemination. The collection and publication of translational evidence relevant to implementation remain insufficient. Multiple frameworks and tools are available to help fill this evidence gap and enable evaluation and better understanding of the barriers to, facilitators of, and readiness for intervention implementation. More work to incorporate implementation science into the design, monitoring, and evaluation of interventions will be important to the continuing advancement of improvements in dementia care.

CONCLUSION: Interventions that demonstrate efficacy in a clinical trial or other controlled research setting need to be adapted to local settings, tailored to the targeted populations, and monitored and evaluated to assess their effectiveness when translated to an uncontrolled clinical or community setting and to guide adjustments to the implementation process. Some adaptations of and changes to the implementation context and conditions will undermine effectiveness, and some interventions with efficacy may not work in real-world settings.

CONCLUSION: To inform decisions about whether and under what circumstances to implement and fund an intervention, stakeholders—such as persons living with dementia, care partners and caregivers, health care and long-term services and supports providers, care systems, payers, and policy makers—consider evidence on effectiveness; stakeholder values; and the contexts in which an intervention may be implemented, such as individual characteristics of participants (e.g., stage of dementia, race/ethnicity), organizational structure, workforce, and payment models. Different stakeholders may use different criteria to inform their decisions on the implementation of dementia care interventions.

REFERENCES

Alonso-Coello, P., H. J. Schünemann, J. Moberg, R. Brignardello-Petersen, E. A. Akl, M. Davoli, S. Treweek, R. A. Mustafa, G. Rada, S. Rosenbaum, A. Morelli, G. H. Guyatt, and A. D. Oxman. 2016. GRADE Evidence to Decision (EtD) frameworks: A systematic and transparent approach to making well informed healthcare choices. 1: Introduction. *BMJ* 353:i2016.

Borson, S., J. Chodosh, C. Cordell, B. Kallmyer, M. Boustani, A. Chodos, J. K. Dave, L. Gwyther, S. Reed, D. B. Reuben, S. Stabile, M. Willis-Parker, and W. Thies. 2017. Innovation in care for individuals with cognitive impairment: Can reimbursement policy spread best practices? *Alzheimer's & Dementia* 13(10):1168–1173.

Boustani, M. A., S. Munger, R. Gulati, M. Vogel, R. A. Beck, and C. M. Callahan. 2010. Selecting a change and evaluating its impact on the performance of a complex adaptive health care delivery system. *Clinical Interventions in Aging* 5:141–148.

Boustani, M., C. A. Alder, and C. A. Solid. 2018. Agile implementation: A blueprint for implementing evidence-based healthcare solutions. *Journal of the American Geriatrics Society* 66(7):1372–1376.

Boustani, M., C. A. Alder, C. A. Solid, and D. Reuben. 2019. An alternative payment model to support widespread use of collaborative dementia care models. *Health Affairs* 38(1):54–59.

Bradley, E. H., T. R. Webster, D. Baker, M. Schlesinger, S. K. Inouye, M. C. Barth, K. L. Lapane, D. Lipson, R. Stone, and M. J. Koren. 2004. Translating research into practice: Speeding the adoption of innovative health care programs. *Issue Brief (Commonwealth Fund)* (724):1–12.

Callahan, C. M., D. R. Bateman, S. Wang, and M. A. Boustani. 2018. State of science: Bridging the science-practice gap in aging, dementia and mental health. *Journal of the American Geriatriatric Society* 66(Suppl 1):S28–S35.

Carroll, C., M. Patterson, S. Wood, A. Booth, J. Rick, and S. Balain. 2007. A conceptual framework for implementation fidelity. *Implementation Science* 2(1):40.

Colello, K. J. 2018. *Who pays for long-term services and supports?* Congressional Research Service, August 22. https://fas.org/sgp/crs/misc/IF10343.pdf (accessed January 21, 2021).

Curran, G. M., M. Bauer, B. Mittman, J. M. Pyne, and C. Stetler. 2012. Effectiveness-implementation hybrid designs: Combining elements of clinical effectiveness and implementation research to enhance public health impact. *Medical Care* 50(3):217–226.

Damschroder, L. J., D. C. Aron, R. E. Keith, S. R. Kirsh, J. A. Alexander, and J. C. Lowery. 2009. Fostering implementation of health services research findings into practice: A consolidated framework for advancing implementation science. *Implementation Science* 4(1):50.

Eccles, M. P., and B. S. Mittman. 2006. Welcome to implementation science. *Implementation Science* 1(1):1.

Gitlin, L. N., K. Marx, I. H. Stanley, and N. Hodgson. 2015. Translating evidence-based dementia caregiving interventions into practice: State-of-the-science and next steps. *Gerontologist* 55(2):210–226.

Glasgow, R. E., S. M. Harden, B. Gaglio, B. Rabin, M. L. Smith, G. C. Porter, M. G. Ory, and P. A. Estabrooks. 2019. RE-AIM planning and evaluation framework: Adapting to new science and practice with a 20-year review. *Frontiers in Public Health* 7(64).

Gupta, R., L. Roh, C. Lee, D. Reuben, A. Naeim, J. Wilson, and S. A. Skootsky. 2019. The population health value framework: Creating value by reducing costs of care for patient subpopulations with chronic conditions. *Academic Medicine* 94(9):1337–1342.

IOM (Institute of Medicine). 2013. *Best care at lower cost: The path to continuously learning health care in America*. Washington, DC: The National Academies Press.

IOM. 2015. *Vital signs: Core metrics for health and health care progress*. Washington, DC: The National Academies Press.

Lees Haggerty, K., G. Epstein-Lubow, L. H. Spragens, R. J. Stoeckle, L. C. Evertson, L. A. Jennings, and D. B. Reuben. 2020. Recommendations to improve payment policies for comprehensive dementia care. *Journal of the American Geriatrics Society* 68(11):2478–2485.

Lourida, I., R. A. Abbott, M. Rogers, I. A. Lang, K. Stein, B. Kent, and J. Thompson Coon. 2017. Dissemination and implementation research in dementia care: A systematic scoping review and evidence map. *BMC Geriatrics* 17(1):147.

Moberg, J., A. D. Oxman, S. Rosenbaum, H. J. Schünemann, G. Guyatt, S. Flottorp, C. Glenton, S. Lewin, A. Morelli, G. Rada, P. Alonso-Coello, E. Akl, M. Gulmezoglu, R. A. Mustafa, J. Singh, E. von Elm, J. Vogel, and J. Watine. 2018. The GRADE Evidence to Decision (EtD) framework for health system and public health decisions. *Health Research Policy and Systems* 16(1):45.

Murray, E., S. Treweek, C. Pope, A. MacFarlane, L. Ballini, C. Dowrick, T. Finch, A. Kennedy, F. Mair, C. O'Donnell, B. N. Ong, T. Rapley, A. Rogers, and C. May. 2010. Normalisation process theory: A framework for developing, evaluating and implementing complex interventions. *BMC Medicine* 8(1):63.

NAE (National Academy of Engineering). 2011. *Engineering a learning healthcare system: A look at the future: Workshop summary*. Washington, DC: The National Academies Press.

NASEM (National Academies of Sciences, Engineering, and Medicine). 2016. *Families caring for an aging America*. Washington, DC: The National Academies Press.

NIA (National Institute on Aging). 2018. *Stage model for behavioral intervention development*. https://www.nia.nih.gov/research/dbsr/nih-stage-model-behavioral-intervention-development (accessed August 18, 2020).

NQF (National Quality Forum). 2016. *Quality in home and community-based services to support community living: Addressing gaps in performance measurement*. Washington, DC: National Quality Forum.

Petticrew, M., C. Knai, J. Thomas, E. A. Rehfuess, J. Noyes, A. Gerhardus, J. M. Grimshaw, H. Rutter, and E. McGill. 2019. Implications of a complexity perspective for systematic reviews and guideline development in health decision making. *BMJ Global Health* 4(Suppl 1):e000899.

Proctor, E., H. Silmere, R. Raghavan, P. Hovmand, G. Aarons, A. Bunger, R. Griffey, and M. Hensley. 2011. Outcomes for implementation research: Conceptual distinctions, measurement challenges, and research agenda. *Administration and Policy in Mental Health* 38(2):65–76.

Rogers, E. M. 2003. *Diffusion of innovations*, 5th ed. New York: Free Press.

Rutter, H., N. Savona, K. Glonti, J. Bibby, S. Cummins, D. T. Finegood, F. Greaves, L. Harper, P. Hawe, L. Moore, M. Petticrew, E. Rehfuess, A. Shiell, J. Thomas, and M. White. 2017. The need for a complex systems model of evidence for public health. *The Lancet* 390(10112):2602–2604.

Sohn, H., A. Tucker, O. Ferguson, I. Gomes, and D. Dowdy. 2020. Costing the implementation of public health interventions in resource-limited settings: A conceptual framework. *Implementation Science* 15(1):86.

Teisberg, E., S. Wallace, and S. O'Hara. 2020. Defining and implementing value-based health care: A strategic framework. *Academic Medicine* 95(5).

The Lewin Group. 2018. *Final evaluation report: Testing experience and functional tools in home and community-based services demonstration program*. Centers for Medicare & Medicaid Services. https://www.medicaid.gov/sites/default/files/2019-12/teft-evaluation-final-report.pdf (accessed January 21, 2021).

University of Washington. 2020. *What is implementation science?* https://impsciuw.org/implementation-science/learn/implementation-science-overview (accessed September 8, 2020).

Unützer, J., A. C. Carlo, R. Arao, M. Vredevoogd, J. Fortney, D. Powers, and J. Russo. 2020. Variation in the effectiveness of collaborative care for depression: Does it matter where you get your care? *Health Affairs* 39(11):1943–1950.

Walugembe, D. R., S. Sibbald, M. J. Le Ber, and A. Kothari. 2019. Sustainability of public health interventions: Where are the gaps? *Health Research Policy and Systems* 17(1):8.

WHO (World Health Organization). 2004. *Monitoring and evaluation toolkit: HIV/AIDS, tuberculosis and malaria*. https://www.who.int/malaria/publications/atoz/a85537/en (accessed January 21, 2021).

Woltmann, E. M., R. Whitley, G. J. McHugo, M. Brunette, W. C. Torrey, L. Coots, D. Lynde, and R. E. Drake. 2008. The role of staff turnover in the implementation of evidence-based practices in mental health care. *Psychiatric Services* 59(7):732–737.

5

ASSESSING THE CURRENT STATE OF EVIDENCE

Much is already known about principles that should guide care, supports, and services for persons living with dementia, as well as core components of care that should be provided throughout the course of the condition (see Chapter 2). Unfortunately, many persons living with dementia lack access to or do not receive these core components; nonetheless, further study is not needed to conclude that they should be provided to all. It should be noted, moreover, that at the individual or family level, persons living with dementia, care partners, and caregivers may want to experiment with such pleasurable activities as listening to music that can be tailored to their personal interests and carry little potential harm to see what works for them, knowing this may change as the condition progresses. This report, however, focuses on what is known about the effectiveness of specific care interventions, services, and supports to serve as the basis for decision making about their broad dissemination and implementation and to inform the relative prioritization of interventions that could be helpful but will require resources that are limited.

This chapter begins with a review of the evidence supporting the two types of dementia care interventions for which the Agency for Healthcare Research and Quality (AHRQ) systematic review found sufficient evidence to support conclusions about effectiveness: collaborative care models and a multicomponent intervention for family caregivers (REACH [Resources for Enhancing Alzheimer's Caregiver Health] II and its adaptations). It then examines gaps in and opportunities for improving and expanding the evidence base on other dementia care interventions.

INTERVENTIONS READY FOR IMPLEMENTATION IN REAL-WORLD SETTINGS WITH MONITORING, EVALUATION, QUALITY IMPROVEMENT, AND INFORMATION SHARING

This section first details the committee's approach to assessing the evidence on readiness for broad dissemination and implementation of the above two types of interventions, including application of the GRADE (Grading of Recommendations Assessment, Development and Evaluation) Evidence to Decision (EtD) framework. It then reviews the evidence, drawn, as explained below, not only from the AHRQ systematic review's findings on effectiveness but also from supplemental sources addressing not only effectiveness but also the criteria of the EtD framework.

Approach to Assessing the Evidence on Readiness for Broad Dissemination and Implementation

Ideally, decisions to broadly disseminate and implement interventions for persons living with dementia, care partners, and caregivers would be informed primarily by evidence from multiple large, rigorous randomized controlled trials (RCTs) that tested an intervention in all relevant settings where it was to be provided; included participants from all representative populations; and tested key factors related to successful implementation, such as integration into existing workflows and contextual factors related to the settings in which the intervention was designed to be delivered. However, the AHRQ systematic review found limited such evidence, finding sufficient evidence to draw conclusions about effectiveness for only the two types of interventions noted above—collaborative care models and multicomponent interventions for family caregivers (REACH II and adaptations)—each found to be supported by low-strength evidence of benefit on specific outcomes for persons living with dementia or care partners and caregivers (Butler et al., 2020) (see Box 5-1).

Given the limitations of the evidence base, the AHRQ systematic review was unable to draw conclusions regarding all other interventions examined. According to the authors, "Ultimately, we uncovered very little evidence to support interventions and programs for active, widespread dissemination because evidence was insufficient to draw conclusions about the effects of the vast majority of interventions studied" (Butler et al., 2020, p. ES-3). This does not necessarily mean that those interventions are not helpful for persons living with dementia, care partners, or caregivers. As the authors note,

BOX 5-1
AHRQ Systematic Review: Summary of Findings on Interventions Supported by Low-Strength Evidence of Benefit

Collaborative Care Models

- Collaborative care models [that use multidisciplinary teams to integrate medical and psychosocial approaches to health care for PLWD] (i.e., Care Ecosystems or discrete adaptations of the ACCESS models) may improve PLWD quality of life. (low-strength evidence) This improvement may be very small to small, or it may be larger but concentrated in some not yet identified subgroup of people.
- Collaborative care models (i.e., discrete adaptations of the ACCESS model) may improve system-level markers, including guideline-based quality indicators and reduction in emergency department visits. (low-strength evidence)
- Evidence was insufficient to draw conclusions about all other outcomes for both PLWD and CG/P.

Multicomponent Interventions for Informal Caregivers

- Intensive multicomponent intervention with education, group discussion, in-home and phone support sessions, and caregiver feedback for CG/P support (i.e., discrete adaptations of REACH II), improved CG/P depression at 6 months. (low-strength evidence)
- Evidence was insufficient to draw conclusions about the effect of other forms of multicomponent interventions on PLWD and their CG/P.

NOTES: CG/P = care partners/caregivers; PLWD = persons living with dementia; REACH = Resources for Enhancing Alzheimer's Caregiver Health. Terminology and abbreviations used in this box are those of the AHRQ systematic review and do not necessarily correspond to the terminology used in this report.
SOURCE: Excerpted from Butler et al., 2020, pp. 77, 93.

> Rather, it means that current available evidence cannot yet provide clear answers about which interventions offer consistent benefits. Therefore, the uncertainty of the evidence is too high for us to draw conclusions, at present. Furthermore, when the evidence overall does not find a difference between groups, uncertainty is even higher about whether the lack of difference is truly because the interventions being compared did not differ in effect, or because the studies were designed to detect differences rather than no difference. (Butler et al., 2020, p. 107)

It is important to emphasize that the AHRQ systematic review was designed specifically to inform the question of which interventions, if any, are ready for broad dissemination and implementation, and the review authors made decisions through this lens that inform the interpretation of the review findings and conclusions. The AHRQ systematic review excluded studies judged to be in Stages 0–II of the National Institutes of Health Stage Model for Behavioral Intervention Development (small-sample or pilot studies) and those judged to have high risk of bias (Butler et al., 2020).[1] Stages 0–II describe early-stage research that has not yet included testing of interventions in real-world settings. Excluding studies that have small sample sizes or high risk of bias is standard in systematic reviews. However, exclusion of the heterogeneous category of pilots is important to interpreting the systematic review findings. While many pilots are small and preliminary, the review also excluded some studies that are described by the study authors as pilots although they used relatively large sample sizes (i.e., hundreds of participants), and in some cases were conducted in the community with relatively long follow-up times. An example of such a study is an assessment of the Maximizing Independence at Home (MIND) program in a pilot RCT involving 303 community-dwelling individuals that included two arms, with outcomes being measured at 18 months (Samus et al., 2014). Had the AHRQ review targeted specific interventions in more depth and included research-setting efficacy studies without applying the lens of readiness for dissemination and implementation, the analysis and conclusions might have been different. Because these pilot studies were excluded from the systematic review, it is unknown what portion of them could potentially be informative for determining efficacy and what portion would be excluded because of sample size or quality concerns. Considerations related to the trajectory of development in this field and approaches for developing the evidence base needed to support implementation in the real world are explored later in this chapter and in Chapter 6.

The limitations described above make it challenging to answer the core question that motivated this study of which dementia care interventions, if any, are ready for broad dissemination and implementation. To provide the most complete view of the evidence available to inform decision making in real-world settings, the committee supplemented the AHRQ review findings by applying the GRADE EtD framework and considering supplemental evidence, as described below.

---

[1] Of the 627 unique studies eligible for analysis, 409 were excluded because they had small sample sizes or were pilots, and an additional 218 were assessed as having high risk of bias. Recognizing the challenges of conducting research in this area, the AHRQ systematic review authors set the sample-size criterion generously: studies were excluded only if they had fewer than 10 participants per arm. Similarly, the review authors characterize their approach to assessing risk of bias as "generous, relative to how risk of bias is assessed in more targeted systematic review topics." For example, studies were assessed as having high risk of bias due to attrition only if attrition was greater than 40 percent (Butler et al., 2020, pp. 20, 108).

The findings of the AHRQ systematic review with regard to intervention effectiveness were used to identify the above two types of interventions as potentially ready for broad dissemination and implementation. In addition to effectiveness, however, many factors need to be considered in determining whether broad implementation of an intervention is appropriate. To inform the development of its recommendations on the two types of interventions identified in the systematic review as supported by low-strength evidence of benefit (see Figure 5-1), the committee applied the GRADE EtD framework. As described in Chapter 4, this framework can be used to consider evidence on factors in addition to effectiveness in making and using clinical recommendations, coverage decisions, and health system and public health recommendations and decisions (Alonso-Coello et al., 2016; Moberg et al., 2018). Factors taken into account in the assessment can include the priority of the problem, how substantial the benefits and harms are, the certainty of the evidence, the value of the outcomes to stakeholders, how the intervention or option in question compares with others, resource requirements, cost effectiveness versus comparable options, the impact on health equity, the acceptability of the intervention to stakeholders, and the feasibility of implementation.

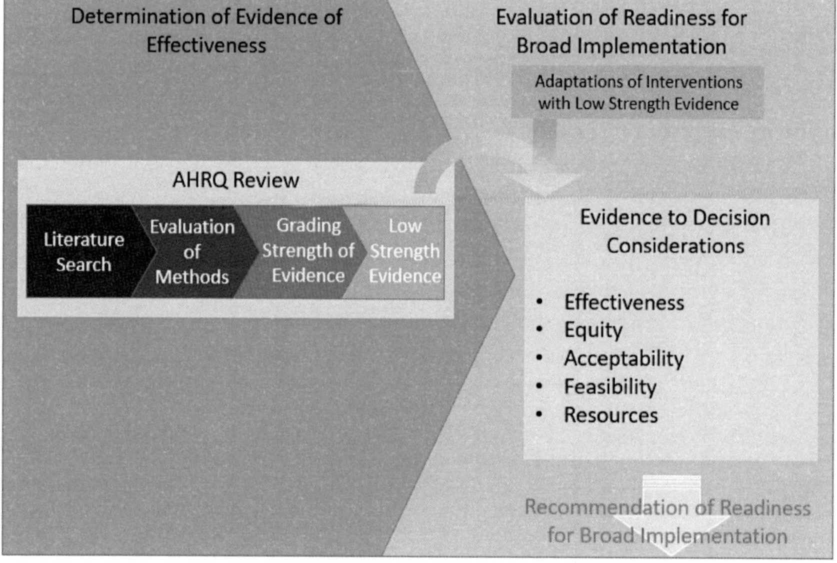

FIGURE 5-1 Framework for the use of evidence to make recommendations regarding the broad implementation of dementia care interventions.
SOURCE: Adapted from NASEM, 2020.

For the EtD assessment, the committee culled available evidence on each criterion from studies that met the AHRQ review criteria for inclusion. The committee also examined evidence in other available published studies on these interventions. In particular, REACH II has been adapted for different populations and implemented in a variety of settings. The AHRQ review authors rated some of these implementation studies as having high risk of bias and excluded others because they used methodologies that failed to meet their inclusion criteria, such as studies with a single pre–posttest. Nevertheless, these studies provide such information as feasibility, equity, and resources required that is important for making decisions regarding implementation in the real world. The committee identified these additional studies by reference mining the studies that met the AHRQ review inclusion criteria, reviewing studies mentioned in the AHRQ review that did not meet the inclusion criteria, conducting PubMed and hand searches, and reviewing the Best Practice Caregiving database and Center for Medicare & Medicaid Innovation (CMMI) evaluations.

Together, these studies provide a rich source of evidence regarding effectiveness beyond the outcomes on which the AHRQ review was able to draw conclusions. Thus, without negating the AHRQ review's conclusions regarding the low strength of evidence or the uncertainties that prevented the review from reaching conclusions on many outcomes, the committee deemed that compiling this comprehensive set of available evidence on effectiveness could be informative for those considering implementing these two types of interventions in a range of settings. Accordingly, the sections below include discussion of trends in intervention benefits across a range of outcomes beyond those for which the AHRQ review was able to draw conclusions. These findings include primary outcomes from individual studies for which the AHRQ review found insufficient evidence to draw a conclusion (often because of inconsistencies in this outcome across studies), primary outcomes not included in the AHRQ review,[2] secondary outcomes mentioned in the AHRQ review, and results from implementation studies that did not meet the AHRQ inclusion criteria. It is important to note that these additional data on effectiveness are provided for descriptive purposes; the committee's conclusions and recommendations rest on the AHRQ review findings and the EtD assessment, as well as on the

---

[2] "For the KQs, we assessed the effects of outcomes using clinically important differences if well-established, but for many outcomes this was not the case. Because of the very wide range of outcomes of interest across the panel of potential interventions, we did not list specific priority outcomes beyond those noted in Table 1.1. For any individual study, we examined no more than five to seven outcomes per PLWD or caregiver population, prioritizing person-centered outcomes, (e.g., quality of life, function, and harms), over intermediate outcomes (e.g., laboratory test values, subscales of outcome measurement tools). Our rationale for this decision is that excessive reporting of outcomes generally happens with the latter type of outcome" (Butler et al., 2020, p. 18).

committee's analysis of the most effective path forward for improving the evidence base for these interventions, as described later in this chapter.

Collaborative Care Models

The AHRQ systematic review identified 13 unique studies of collaborative care models from 32 publications (Butler et al., 2020). Of these 13 studies, 7 were determined to have low or medium risk of bias and proceeded to analysis. These studies report outcomes for persons living with dementia and care partners/caregivers, but the AHRQ review found sufficient evidence to support conclusions only on three outcomes for persons living with dementia. The review found insufficient evidence to support conclusions on the other outcomes for persons living with dementia evaluated in collaborative care interventions, as well as on benefits to care partners/caregivers. Box 5-1, presented earlier, provides the AHRQ summary of findings.

The AHRQ systematic review describes collaborative care models as care delivery interventions that use multidisciplinary teams integrating both medical and psychosocial approaches to the care of persons living with dementia (Butler et al., 2020). Collaborative care models may include individuals with multiple comorbidities, as is the case for both the ACCESS and Care Ecosystem models (Boustani et al., 2019; Possin et al., 2019; Vickrey et al., 2006). This section provides an overview of the AHRQ review's analysis of evidence on collaborative care models, examines limitations of the evidence and the analysis, and applies the GRADE EtD framework to inform discussion of the readiness of these models for broad dissemination and implementation.[3] Box 5-2 provides a brief description of those collaborative care models that were included in the AHRQ analytic set and demonstrated benefit on at least one outcome.

Summary of AHRQ Findings on the Effectiveness of Collaborative Care Models

As described in Box 5-2, the seven studies of collaborative care models included in the AHRQ systematic review's analytic set examined six different model interventions. The three outcomes for persons living with dementia for which the AHRQ review found sufficient evidence to draw conclusions were (1) quality of life, (2) quality indicators, and (3) emergency room visits. Box 5-1, presented earlier, provides the AHRQ descrip-

[3] For the purposes of this assessment, benefit as reported here is based on statistical significance, consistent with the AHRQ systematic review approach. This was extracted from the AHRQ systematic review for those studies included in its analytic set, and from the results reported in the original study for those studies not included in the analytic set.

BOX 5-2
Description of Selected Collaborative Care Models Analyzed by the AHRQ Systematic Review

The collaborative care interventions analyzed by the Agency for Healthcare Research and Quality (AHRQ) systematic review share multiple components, including coordination of services through a care manager, the development of care plans, case tracking, and collaboration with care providers. This box includes only those interventions for which a benefit was found on at least one outcome.

ACCESS Model: A dementia management program administered by care managers with referrals to health care organization and community agency care managers in two Southern California communities (Chodosh et al., 2015; Vickrey et al., 2006).

Care Ecosystem: A telephone-based dementia management program delivered by centralized collaborative care teams in California, Iowa, and Nebraska (Possin et al., 2019).

Central Union for the Welfare of the Aged in Helsinki: An individualized care and services program managed by family care coordinators for persons living with dementia and their spouses in Helsinki, Finland (Eloniemi-Sulkava et al., 2009).

Dementia Care Management: An individualized dementia management program delivered through the existing health care and social service system in Germany (Thyrian et al., 2017).

Indiana University/Purdue University Model: A collaborative care management program delivered by primary care physicians and geriatric nurse practitioners in Indiana (Callahan et al., 2006).*

Partners in Dementia Care: A coaching model led by care coordinators and care coordinator assistants in health care and community service organizations in Boston and Houston (Bass et al., 2013).

---

* The Indiana University/Purdue University collaborative care model, while no longer in use, helped inform the design of an ongoing collaborative care intervention, the Aging Brain Care Medical Home (Callahan et al., 2011). While the results of the Aging Brain Care Medical Home have been reported in various studies, they did not meet the AHRQ review's inclusion criteria.

tion of this intervention category and a summary of the review findings. Findings for persons living with dementia and for care partners/caregivers are discussed in turn below.

Findings for persons living with dementia The AHRQ review evaluated the effect of collaborative care interventions on seven outcomes for persons living with dementia: quality of life, neuropsychiatric symptoms, function, depression, quality indicators, emergency room visits, and nursing home placement (Butler et al., 2020). At least one study reported evidence of benefit for quality of life, neuropsychiatric symptoms, quality indicators, emergency room visits, and nursing home placement. The AHRQ review found no benefit for function or depression in persons living with dementia.

The AHRQ review's analytic set for collaborative care included four studies that evaluated quality of life in persons living with dementia. Of these, two observed benefit: a study of the ACCESS model (Vickrey et al., 2006) and a study of the Care Ecosystem model (Possin et al., 2019). The study of the ACCESS model reported benefit at 18 months follow-up and that of the Care Ecosystem model at 12 months. Two other studies evaluated in the AHRQ review found no benefit for quality of life in persons living with dementia (Chodosh et al., 2015; Thyrian et al., 2017). The conclusion of the AHRQ review was that there was low-strength evidence that collaborative care models improved quality of life in persons living with dementia (Butler et al., 2020). Despite the mixed findings for this outcome, the weighting of larger pragmatic trials in the analysis enabled the AHRQ review to reach this conclusion about low-strength evidence.

One study was included in the AHRQ review's analytic set for the effects of collaborative care on neuropsychiatric symptoms. For the Indiana University/Purdue University collaborative care model, benefit was observed for neuropsychiatric symptoms in persons living with dementia at 12 months follow-up (Callahan et al., 2006). However, this was a relatively small, explanatory study, and the AHRQ review found this evidence insufficient to support a conclusion regarding the effectiveness of collaborative care models for reducing neuropsychiatric symptoms in persons living with dementia.

Two studies assessing quality indicators were included in the AHRQ review's analytic set on collaborative care. Both of these studies evaluated the ACCESS model, and both reported benefit for quality indicators as measured by adherence to dementia care guidelines at an average of 22.5 months (Vickrey et al., 2006) and either 6 months or 12 months follow-up (Chodosh et al., 2015). Given these findings, the AHRQ review concluded that there was low-strength evidence that collaborative care models improved quality indicators.

The AHRQ review's analytic set for collaborative care models included one study that evaluated emergency room visits. This study assessed the Care Ecosystem model, and observed benefit for decreasing emergency room visits for persons living with dementia during 12 months of follow-up (Possin et al., 2019). While this was the only collaborative care study evaluating emergency room visits, AHRQ's analysis was weighted for larger pragmatic trials, leading to the AHRQ review's conclusion that there was low-strength evidence that collaborative care models decreased emergency room visits for persons living with dementia.

The analytic set for collaborative care included three studies assessing nursing home placement for persons living with dementia. The study of the collaborative care model of the Central Union for the Welfare of the Aged in Helsinki reported benefit for nursing home placement at 1.6 years, but not at 2 years (Eloniemi-Sulkava et al., 2009). The other two studies included in the AHRQ review's analysis found no benefit for nursing home placement (Callahan et al., 2006; Thyrian et al., 2017). The AHRQ review determined that there was insufficient evidence to draw a conclusion on the benefit of collaborative care for nursing home placement.

Two studies included in the AHRQ analytic set assessed the effects of collaborative care models on the function of persons living with dementia. Neither of these two studies reported a benefit for function (Callahan et al., 2006; Thyrian et al., 2017).

The AHRQ review included one study evaluating depression among persons living with dementia in the analytic set for collaborative care. This study found no benefit of the collaborative care model for depression (Callahan et al., 2006).

Findings for care partners and caregivers The AHRQ review's analytic set for collaborative care models included studies evaluating five outcomes for care partners and caregivers: quality of life, strain, depression, self-efficacy, and quality measures (Butler et al., 2020). At least one study reported benefit for strain, depression, and quality measures. The AHRQ review found no benefit for quality of life or self-efficacy in care partners and caregivers.

Of the studies in the AHRQ review analytic set that evaluated the effect of collaborative care on care partner and caregiver strain, benefit was observed for both the Care Ecosystem model (Possin et al., 2019) and the Dementia Care Management model (Thyrian et al., 2017) at 12 months follow-up. The other studies included in the analytic set found no benefit for care partner and caregiver strain (Bass et al., 2013; Chodosh et al., 2015; Vickrey et al., 2006). The AHRQ review determined that this inconsistent evidence was insufficient to draw a conclusion on the effects of collaborative care models on care partner and caregiver strain.

The analytic set for collaborative care included three studies evaluating care partner and caregiver depression. Among these three studies, the Care Ecosystem model was the only one for which benefit was observed, having improved care partner and caregiver depression at 12 months follow-up. The other two studies found no benefit for this outcome (Bass et al., 2013; Callahan et al., 2006). Given this evidence, the AHRQ review found that there was insufficient evidence to draw a conclusion on the effect of collaborative care on care partner and caregiver depression.

One study included in the analytic set for collaborative care assessed quality measures. This study of Partners in Dementia Care observed benefit for certain indicators at 6 months follow-up, including unmet needs of care partners and caregivers and use of care partner and caregiver support services, but no benefit for the number of unpaid helpers that assisted with the care of the person living with dementia (Bass et al., 2013).[4] The AHRQ review determined that the evidence was insufficient to draw a conclusion regarding the effects of collaborative care models on quality measures.

The AHRQ review included one study evaluating care partner and caregiver quality of life in the analytic set for collaborative care. This study did not demonstrate benefit for quality of life in care partners and caregivers (Vickrey et al., 2006).

The collaborative care analytic set included one study that measured care partner and caregiver self-efficacy, but it found no benefit for this outcome (Possin et al., 2019).

In addition to the outcomes assessed in the AHRQ review, at 18 months, caregiver participants in ACCESS were more likely to report confidence in caregiving and caregiving mastery, better social support, and receipt of adequate help with patients' problem behaviors and such services as respite care or home health aide services (Vickrey et al., 2006).

Findings for related interventions Several interventions that share features with collaborative care models, including several identified in the AHRQ systematic review in categories other than collaborative care, have been implemented in various settings. These related interventions include programs that restructured the delivery of care through care management teams from a centralized hub (Amjad et al., 2018) or within a specific health care system (Jennings et al., 2020; LaMantia et al., 2015), as well as case management programs designed to help coordinate care and services for persons living with dementia and their care partners/caregivers (Chien and Lee, 2008). These interventions either did not meet the AHRQ systematic review's inclusion criteria or were found to have insufficient evidence for the review to draw a conclusion about their effectiveness.

Limitations of the evidence The AHRQ review aggregated results across different interventions in the collaborative care category to draw conclusions regarding particular outcomes. This approach was not designed to distinguish effectiveness among interventions within a category, a limitation

[4] A translation of Partners in Dementia Care implemented in two sites in Ohio, evaluated with a quasi-experimental, pre–post design, also showed benefit for a decrease in embarrassment about memory problems and unmet needs for persons living with dementia (Bass et al., 2019). The study also found benefit for care partners and caregivers for decreased lack of caregiving confidence and unmet needs.

exacerbated by the lack of common outcome measures (discussed further in Chapter 6). As an illustrative example, studies of four different collaborative care models assessed caregiver burden, with two showing benefit and two showing no effect. Because of this inconsistency across studies, the AHRQ review judged this evidence insufficient to support a conclusion regarding the effect of collaborative care models on caregiver burden. In contrast, the effect on number of emergency room visits was assessed for only one model (Care Ecosystem), and a benefit was reported. In this case, the AHRQ review was able to draw a conclusion based on a single study because it was a large pragmatic study. However, the frequency of inconsistent findings across outcomes that were studied for more than one collaborative care model raises questions about whether similar inconsistencies would have been found had more than one study assessed the emergency room visit outcome. To reflect the AHRQ analytic approach and the complex set of evidence analyzed, and to avoid implying greater certainty about specific models than is warranted by the evidence and the approach to its review, the committee followed the AHRQ analytic approach in examining collaborative care models as an intervention category.

Additional Evidence on Effectiveness

Several collaborative care interventions for which no studies met the AHRQ review inclusion criteria were assessed in CMMI evaluations. The two interventions that had sufficient data enabling CMMI to perform a rigorous analysis were the Aging Brain Care Medical Home program and the University of California, Los Angeles (UCLA), Alzheimer's and Dementia Care program (NORC at the University of Chicago, 2016). Analyzing 3 years of claims data, the CMMI evaluation found no benefit for utilization or cost outcomes for the Aging Brain Care Medical Home participants living with dementia. However, a qualitative analysis of participant focus groups and interviews reported that participants and their care partners and caregivers had improved quality of life and quality of care, and decreased stress, although this finding was not reported by condition, and more than half of the program participants were not living with dementia.

The CMMI evaluation of the UCLA Alzheimer's and Dementia Care program reported a decrease in hospitalizations for ambulatory care–sensitive conditions and in 30-day readmissions for persons living with dementia (NORC at the University of Chicago, 2016). The study of the intervention also reported a decreased risk of persons living with dementia being admitted to long-term care facilities. The cost of care for persons living with dementia who were enrolled in the program was less than that for the comparison group, with a cost savings of $605 per patient per quarter (90% confidence interval: $120, $1,090). A qualitative analysis of participant focus groups reported that persons living with dementia and care partners and caregivers reported an improvement in quality of life and quality of care.

GRADE Evidence to Decision Framework

This section describes available evidence for the criteria of the GRADE EtD framework for the four collaborative care interventions for which positive results were reported for at least one outcome and that were implemented within the United States: ACCESS, Care Ecosystem, the Indiana University/Purdue University model, and Partners in Dementia Care. Two of the collaborative care models for which effectiveness evidence is described above—Central Union for the Welfare of the Aged in Helsinki and the Dementia Care Management program in Germany—were implemented in contexts very different from that of the United States, so that data on such criteria as feasibility and cost would not be applicable.

Equity Collaborative care models have been implemented in racially and ethnically diverse populations spanning various geographic areas. It is important to note, however, that these models have been studied primarily in Black, Hispanic or Latino, and white populations, with less recruitment of individuals of other racial and ethnic groups, such as Asian Americans and American Indians.

The ACCESS trials were designed to be delivered in English or Spanish (Chodosh et al., 2015; Vickrey et al., 2006). Whereas the initial ACCESS intervention drew on a largely white population (Vickrey et al., 2006), another iteration of ACCESS was carried out in a low-income Latino community, and the majority of participants were Hispanic or Latino (Chodosh et al., 2015). The ACCESS program has been implemented in persons living with various types of dementia, including Alzheimer's and vascular dementias, and along the spectrum of severity, with the original trial enrolling mainly individuals with mild and moderate dementia (Vickrey et al., 2006) and an adaptation comprising primarily persons living with moderate and severe dementia symptoms (Chodosh et al., 2015). The ACCESS program also has been implemented in populations of persons living with dementia and care partners/caregivers with less than a high school education (Chodosh et al., 2015; Vickrey et al., 2006), and one study reported that the ACCESS program decreased disparities in quality of care among care partners/caregivers with lower educational attainment (Brown et al., 2013). However, the requirement of phone access to participate in the intervention could pose a barrier to equal access, as some caregivers concerned about limited phone minutes would not respond to calls from program staff (Chodosh et al., 2015).

The Care Ecosystem program was delivered in English, Spanish, or Cantonese (Possin et al., 2019) to participants that identified as Asian

American, Black, Hispanic or Latino, white, or other/mixed race. Participants resided in urban and rural settings across California, Nebraska, and Iowa. About half of the persons living with dementia participating in the intervention had mild symptoms, and persons with moderate and severe dementia each constituted about one-quarter of the participants. The Care Ecosystem model was implemented successfully in a population that included individuals with less than a high school education and with low annual income. While the reliance on phone and Internet access for delivery of the intervention may disproportionately exclude older, rural-dwelling, individuals with lower educational attainment and low-income individuals—groups with lower Internet use (Pew Research Center, 2019a)—the Care Ecosystem model leverages telemedicine to connect individuals in resource-poor areas with specialized dementia care (Possin et al., 2019).

The Indiana University/Purdue University collaborative care model was delivered in an urban Indianapolis health care system that serves low-income individuals, as well as the Indianapolis Veterans Affairs Medical Center (Callahan et al., 2006). Of the persons living with dementia who participated in the intervention, half identified as Black, two-thirds were Medicaid recipients, most had multiple chronic comorbid conditions, and the average years of education attained was approximately 9. The intervention was delivered exclusively in English, and excluded individuals without phone access and persons living with dementia who did not have a consenting caregiver or care partner.

Partners in Dementia Care is an intervention available to veterans living with dementia who receive their primary care from the U.S. Department of Veterans Affairs (VA) and its care partners and caregivers (Bass et al., 2013, 2014, 2015, 2019; Judge et al., 2011; Shrestha et al., 2011). The intervention has been delivered in geographically distinct areas, including Massachusetts, Ohio, and Texas. Between 16 and 21 percent of veterans in the studies of this intervention identified as racial or ethnic minorities. Participants represented a wide range of dementia severity, as well as diversity in levels of educational attainment. Nearly all of the veterans living with dementia were male, and nearly all of the care partners and caregivers were female.

Acceptability The ACCESS intervention has demonstrated some level of acceptability for various stakeholder groups. More than 75 percent of participants remained enrolled in the intervention 6 months after enrollment, although the intervention staff initially experienced difficulties in recruiting dyads to participate (Chodosh et al., 2015). Additionally, the coordination between health care systems and community organizations reduced duplication of effort for dementia care professionals, which may help reduce costs (Vickrey et al., 2006).

Participants in the Care Ecosystem intervention reported high levels of satisfaction with the program. Seventy-eight percent of caregivers said they were satisfied or very satisfied with the services provided, and 97 percent of caregivers indicated that they would recommend the program to another caregiver (Possin et al., 2019).

At the end of the 12-month intervention, 83 percent of the care partners and caregivers that participated in the Indiana University/Purdue University model rated the primary care received by the individual living with dementia in whose care they were involved as very good or excellent (Callahan et al., 2006).

In a survey of the Partners in Dementia Care care coordinators, respondents described the acceptance and use of the program by persons living with dementia and their families as a moderate challenge to implementation (Judge et al., 2011). Respondents also found physician participation to be a minor difficulty.

Feasibility Collaborative care models tend to leverage existing health care and community resources, a feature that may make implementing such models across diverse settings more feasible.

The authors of the ACCESS intervention emphasize that the ability of the program to link patients and caregivers with existing community resources facilitates the adaptation of ACCESS to other settings (Vickrey et al., 2006). The in-home arm of one of the ACCESS studies encountered difficulties with fully implementing the home contacts, with the average number of in-person contacts received being just one rather than the planned six (Chodosh et al., 2015). In addition, staff involved in that trial offered suggestions for addressing issues they encountered with recruitment, especially among underserved populations, which may be useful to those considering the implementation of this intervention. These suggestions included hiring intervention staff from the target community, who would help build trust and anticipate challenges, and leveraging community resources, such as religious institutions, for outreach.

The Care Ecosystem intervention has several features that allow for greater scalability. The intervention does not require face-to-face visits, enabling dementia care to be provided to those in rural or resource-poor settings (Possin et al., 2019). In addition, the use of intervention staff as first points of contact allowed dementia specialists to attend to work that required their expertise. The intervention also can be delivered from a centralized hub to participants across large geographic areas and different health systems or within a single health care system.

The Indiana University/Purdue University model is centered in primary care practices, which takes advantage of the fact that primary care settings are where most older adults receive medical care (Callahan et al., 2006).

However, the authors note that the financial costs and practice design requirements of implementing this intervention may be impractical for many primary care practices.

Partners in Dementia Care leverages the skill sets and resources of health care in VA medical centers and of community organizations in local chapters of the Alzheimer's Association or Area Agency on Aging (Bass et al., 2015, 2019; Judge et al., 2011; Shrestha et al., 2011). While the intervention has been tested only in veterans receiving care from the VA, the VA operates the largest health care system in the United States, and the intervention has been translated to various VA medical centers and community partnerships (Bass et al., 2019). The study authors describe these partnerships as successful, noting that neither organization was overly burdened and that intervention activities were equally distributed between the VA medical centers and community partners (Shrestha et al., 2011).

The feasibility of implementing collaborative care models has also been demonstrated in additional interventions for dementia and for other diseases. A systematic review (Dham et al., 2017) and a meta-analysis (Archer et al., 2012) found that such models were effective interventions for adults with various psychiatric conditions. A narrative review of emerging collaborative care interventions for dementia also describes a general finding of feasibility and sustainability for the interventions across settings, as well as responsiveness to the needs of health care systems (Heintz et al., 2020). These authors urge ongoing research and the use of implementation science to advance and improve collaborative care models. At the same time, the optimism surrounding the feasibility of these models may be tempered by the fact that existing health care models are resistant to change, and that broad implementation of the models will require the commitment of intervention staff, health care administrators, payers, and regulatory bodies.

Resources In a cost analysis of the ACCESS intervention, the start-up cost is estimated as $70,256 and ongoing intervention costs at $118 per patient per month (Duru et al., 2009). In another study, the estimated cost of an ACCESS adaptation is $358 per patient per month for the in-home intervention and $216 for the telephone-based intervention, with intervention costs taking salaries, mileage, and organizational overhead into account (Chodosh et al., 2015). It is not clear whether the differences in intervention costs between these two ACCESS studies is due to differences in how the calculations were performed. In the Duru and colleagues (2009) study, average monthly health care costs, including service costs, out-of-pocket expenditures, costs of family caregiving, and spending for end-of-life care, are estimated as $6,479 for intervention participants and $6,381 for the usual care control. However, health care costs were higher for the control group than for the intervention group when costs of end-of-life care were excluded. In the Chodosh and colleagues (2015) study, the costs related to health service utilization over a 1-year period are calculated as $5,595 for the in-home intervention and $7,761 for the telephone-based intervention. The authors do not discuss potential reasons for the difference in costs between the in-home and telephone-based implementations.

The cost of the Care Ecosystem intervention averaged from $202 to $762 per person living with dementia per month, depending on the location and stage of the intervention (Rosa et al., 2019). The calculation of intervention costs includes personnel, supplies, equipment, training, and facilities. Overall, intervention costs decreased as caseloads for intervention staff increased as a result of the efficiencies of scaling the program to cover more participants. A CMMI evaluation of Care Ecosystem observed slightly lower (5 percent) Medicare expenditures for program participants compared with control participants, although this difference may not be a result of the program (Gilman et al., 2020).

There is no formal cost analysis for the Indiana University/Purdue University collaborative care model (Callahan et al., 2006). However, the study authors estimate the cost of the care manager to be $1,000 per patient annually, with a caseload of 75 patients. The authors suggest that with the cost savings from a reduction in neuropsychiatric symptoms, a cost analysis may find the intervention to be cost-beneficial.

A cost analysis of the Partners in Dementia Care intervention estimates the cost of the intervention to range from $780 to $960 per dyad per year (Morgan et al., 2015). Costs of the intervention include, among others, staff salaries, equipment, supplies, and training. Total health care costs per intervention participant, including such expenditures as inpatient and outpatient care and pharmacy costs, were $1,006 (standard deviation $9,607) higher for the intervention group than for a control group when adjusted for baseline characteristics. Total health care costs for the intervention and control groups demonstrated a great degree of variability and were highly skewed.

Conclusion Regarding Collaborative Care Models

As a whole, the evidence supporting collaborative care models is encouraging. These interventions have been studied in multiple and diverse populations and with individuals along the spectrum of disease severity. While these interventions have been disseminated and used in relatively limited ways to date, some evidence related to acceptability, feasibility, and resources is available to inform implementation.

> CONCLUSION: *Collaborative care models—which use multidisciplinary teams integrating both medical and psychosocial*

approaches to the care of persons living with dementia—have demonstrated some effectiveness under clinical trial conditions and are already being implemented in care settings with promising results. These interventions are ready for the next stage of field testing to support their widespread adaptation to and adoption in the variety of settings where people seek dementia care. Those efforts will enhance understanding and information dissemination with respect to key factors in addition to effectiveness that are important for deciding whether and how to implement an intervention, such as determining the workforce and space needed; testing payment models and integration into workflow; and ensuring adaptations for different populations (e.g., racial/ethnic groups) and settings (e.g., rural areas).

A Multicomponent Intervention for Family Caregivers: REACH II and Its Adaptations

The AHRQ systematic review identified 22 unique studies of multicomponent interventions for care partners and caregivers, 7 of which were rated as having a low or medium risk of bias and were included in the analysis (Butler et al., 2020). These 7 studies examined three different multicomponent interventions. The AHRQ review found sufficient evidence to draw conclusions about one of these multicomponent interventions (REACH II), but not about the other two. Box 5-1, presented earlier, provides the AHRQ summary of findings.

The three multicomponent interventions analyzed by the AHRQ review comprised different components; the common element of interventions in this category is simply having multiple components. Because the question at hand is what specific interventions are supported by sufficient evidence to be considered ready for broad dissemination and implementation, the committee limited further exploration of this category to the one intervention found to be supported by low-strength evidence of effectiveness in the AHRQ review.

This section provides an overview of available evidence on REACH II and its adaptations, examines limitations of the evidence, and applies the GRADE EtD framework to inform a discussion of the readiness of this intervention for broad dissemination and implementation. Box 5-3 describes the components of REACH II and related adaptations for different populations.

BOX 5-3
A Multicomponent Intervention for Family Caregivers: REACH II and Related Adaptations

Description of Components

Problem solving: Identification of strategies to implement, addressing self-care, problem behaviors, or social support.

Skills training: Techniques for addressing self-care, problem behaviors, or social support.

Stress management: Well-being activities implemented to reduce stress.

Support groups: Telephone-based space for caregivers to discuss experiences with one another.

Provision of information: Information resources made available to caregivers.

Didactic instruction: Educational material discussed with caregivers.

Role playing: Active techniques used to practice implementation of problem-solving strategies.

Description of Adaptations for Different Populations

REACH OUT: Quasi-experimental pre–post evaluation of a condensed REACH II intervention delivered through a social service agency in Alabama (Burgio et al., 2009).

REACH VA: Quasi-experimental pre–post evaluation of the standard REACH II intervention delivered in U.S. Department of Veterans Affairs (VA) Medical Center Home-Based Primary Care programs across the United States (Nichols et al., 2011).

REACH-TX: Quasi-experimental pre–post evaluation of a condensed, risk-tailored REACH II intervention delivered through a community agency and local Alzheimer's Association partnership in North Central Texas (Cho et al., 2019; Stevens et al., 2012).

REACH II (North Texas): Quasi-experimental pre–post evaluation of the standard REACH II intervention delivered through a community organization and local Alzheimer's Association partnership in North Texas (Lykens et al., 2014).

REACH II via videophone: Randomized controlled trial evaluating a condensed REACH II intervention delivered primarily by videoconference technology in Miami, Florida (Czaja et al., 2013).

continued

BOX 5-3 Continued

REACH-HK: Quasi-experimental pre–post evaluation of the standard REACH II intervention delivered through an Alzheimer's foundation and local social services administration partnership in Hong Kong (Cheung et al., 2014).

Community REACH: Quasi-experimental pre–post evaluation of the standard REACH II intervention with greater emphasis on telephone sessions, delivered through a nonprofit home health organization in southern Florida (Czaja et al., 2018; Luchsinger et al., 2018).

DE-REACH: Randomized controlled trial evaluating a condensed REACH II intervention without telephone support sessions, delivered through the German health care system (Berwig et al., 2017).

Summary of AHRQ Findings on the Effectiveness of REACH II

The AHRQ systematic review found low-strength evidence that REACH II improved care partner/caregiver depression at 6 months (Butler et al., 2020). Other outcomes examined included care partner/caregiver health, stress, and strain, but the review was unable to draw conclusions about these outcomes because the definition, measurement, and reporting of outcomes varied so widely. The AHRQ REACH II findings were based on three RCTs. The original trial studied the intervention in a population that was one-third Black or African American, one-third white or Caucasian, and one-third Hispanic or Latino (Belle et al., 2006). That study reported that the intervention was effective for decreasing the prevalence of caregiver depression. While the prevalence of caregiver depression decreased across racial and ethnic groups, only white caregivers exhibited a benefit in the decrease in depression when the results for the three groups were disaggregated. A German adaptation observed a decrease in caregiver depression (Berwig et al., 2017), a finding based on the psychological component of health-related quality of life as measured by the SF-12, which has been used as a tool to detect depressive disorders (Vilagut et al., 2013). And a study with Hispanic caregivers that compared the community-based REACH OUT adaptation with another intervention, the New York University Caregiver Intervention, found no difference between those two interventions and no change in caregiver depression from baseline (Luchsinger et al., 2018).

In addition to the low-strength evidence on reduction in caregiver depression, the AHRQ review identified a reduction in caregiver strain associated with the REACH II adaptation DE-REACH (Berwig et al., 2017). However, this reduction was limited to Black caregivers in one of the studies (Belle et al., 2006). REACH OUT improved caregiver strain compared with baseline but not with the comparator intervention (Luchsinger et al., 2018). Ultimately, the available evidence was insufficient to draw a conclusion on the effectiveness of REACH II in reducing caregiver strain (Butler et al., 2020).

REACH II has been studied in and adapted for diverse populations to a greater extent than is usual in the field, as discussed in greater depth below. In addition, the AHRQ review concluded that there was "more development along the NIH [National Institutes of Health] Stage Model in this set than in most other intervention categories. This literature set demonstrates growth over time toward the development of both pragmatic trials as well as dissemination/implementation research" (Butler et al., 2020, p. 78).

Additional Evidence on Effectiveness

In additional studies of REACH II and its adaptations, study authors have observed a range of beneficial outcomes. With the exception of caregiver depression, the AHRQ review found insufficient evidence to support conclusions about these outcomes. The additional studies described in this section were not included in the AHRQ review analytic set, in many cases because they used an ineligible study design, such as a single pre–posttest. Their findings are described briefly here to illustrate the trends in benefits observed with this intervention.

The results of these studies suggest benefits for reductions in caregiver strain or stress (Burgio et al., 2009; Cheung et al., 2014; Cho et al., 2019; Czaja et al., 2013, 2018; Lykens et al., 2014; Nichols et al., 2011; Stevens et al., 2012), caregiver depression (Burgio et al., 2009; Cheung et al., 2014; Cho et al., 2019; Czaja et al., 2018; Lykens et al., 2014; Nichols et al., 2011), challenging behaviors of the persons living with dementia (Berwig et al., 2017; Burgio et al., 2009; Cheung et al., 2014; Cho et al., 2019; Nichols et al., 2011; Stevens et al., 2012), caregiver frustration or bother (Cheung et al., 2014; Czaja et al., 2018; Nichols et al., 2011), and physical symptoms of psychiatric conditions (Berwig et al., 2017). Studies of REACH II adaptations and implementations also reported improvements in self-reported social support (Burgio et al., 2009; Cho et al., 2019; Czaja et al., 2013, 2018), self-reported caregiver health (Burgio et al., 2009), caregiver reactions to challenging behaviors (Berwig et al., 2017; Czaja et al., 2018), positive aspects of caregiving (Burgio et al., 2009; Cheung et al., 2014; Czaja et al., 2013), and safety of persons living with dementia (Stevens et al., 2012).

Application of the GRADE Evidence to Decision Framework

This section reviews available evidence for the GRADE EtD domains related to REACH II and its adaptations.

Equity REACH II and its adaptations have been carried out in racially and ethnically diverse study populations within the United States, including Asian American, Black, Hispanic or Latino, and white caregivers (Belle et al., 2006; Burgio et al., 2009; Cho et al., 2019; Czaja et al., 2013, 2018; Lykens et al., 2014), and the role of demographic characteristics in moderating the effectiveness of REACH II has been described in detail (Lee et al., 2010). However, much of the research on REACH II has been focused on Black, Hispanic or Latino, and white participants, with other racial and ethnic groups, such as Asian Americans and American Indians, representing small proportions of the populations studied. Of note, REACH II, REACH-TX, REACH II (North Texas), and REACH II via videophone were designed to be delivered in English or Spanish (Belle et al., 2006; Cho et al., 2019; Czaja et al., 2013; Lykens et al., 2014). Several of the REACH II iterations have been implemented successfully in low-income communities or with low-income participants (Belle et al., 2006; Cheung et al., 2014; Czaja et al., 2018). Many REACH II interventions require the use of a cellphone interface, which could potentially preclude the involvement of some caregivers, especially those aged 65 and older, who are less likely than those under age 65 to own a cellphone (Pew Research Center, 2019b). On the other hand, this feature could be helpful for adapting to the current environment in which many activities are being carried out remotely because of the COVID-19 pandemic.

An analysis of the results of REACH II according to racial and ethnic groups observed that the intervention improved quality of life for white and Hispanic or Latino family caregivers, but for Black caregivers, quality of life improved only for those who were caring for a spouse (Belle et al., 2006). The benefit observed for Hispanic or Latino caregivers may be explained in part by the intervention's linguistic and cultural adaptation to this community, which has typically had less access to community services and resources. In the REACH OUT adaptation, white and urban-dwelling caregivers reported a greater reduction in strain relative to Black and rural-dwelling caregivers, respectively (Burgio et al., 2009). Additionally, Black caregivers experienced a larger improvement in positive aspects of caregiving compared with their white counterparts. The REACH II via videophone adaptation was reported to decrease strain for Hispanic but not Black caregivers, although the authors posit that this finding may be due to lower levels of strain among Black participants at baseline (Czaja et al., 2013). In REACH-TX, both young and Black caregivers were more likely to be lost to follow-up compared with other groups, and the authors suggest that strategies for addressing this disparity should be explored (Cho et al., 2019).

Acceptability The REACH II intervention and its adaptations appear to have broad acceptability for participants, intervention staff, and the systems in which the intervention is implemented. Nine hospital units and six clinic care teams were targeted by intervention staff to implement the REACH-TX intervention, and all agreed to participate (Stevens et al., 2012). Only 44 percent of enrolled caregivers completed follow-up. Of these, 82 percent said the services offered were helpful, and 93 percent were satisfied with the quality of those services. Moreover, all participating caregivers reported satisfaction with the information provided and the phone contacts from intervention staff. In a satisfaction survey of the 77 percent of caregivers who completed 6-months' follow-up for Community REACH, 96 percent said that they had benefited from the intervention (Czaja et al., 2018); 93 percent reported that it had made their life easier, and 61 percent agreed that it had improved the life of the person living with dementia. In a REACH II adaptation using videophones, 82 percent of caregivers reported that the intervention was helpful, and 85 percent reported that the support groups were valuable (Czaja et al., 2013). In the REACH OUT adaptation, of the 87 percent of enrolled caregivers that provided responses, 99 percent and 98 percent were satisfied with the type and quality of the intervention, respectively (Burgio et al., 2009). Adherence to the intervention tended to be high, with 95 percent of caregivers receiving all the treatment components during at least one session of the intervention. Similarly, 81 percent of caregivers enrolled in DE-REACH completed at least 10 of 12 sessions (Berwig et al., 2017). Of the 83 percent of caregivers enrolled in REACH-HK who completed follow-up, 92 percent said they would recommend the intervention to other caregivers (Cheung et al., 2014), and all participants in the Community REACH adaptation who completed follow-up said they would recommend it to others (Czaja et al., 2018).

Intervention staff also have reported high levels of satisfaction with REACH II interventions. Case managers for REACH OUT all agreed that they perceived the intervention to be helpful to participants (Burgio et al., 2009). However, many of these same case managers described feeling constrained by time, primarily because the session duration and number of sessions were insufficient to enable them to fully understand and address caregiver concerns, and other aspects of the intervention were time consuming.

Feasibility A number of adaptations of the REACH II intervention have been implemented in community settings, in the VA system, and in various locations around the United States and globally (see Box 5-3 presented earlier). This range of settings provides evidence of the feasibility of adapting the REACH II intervention to suit different settings and cultures and to fit within existing community organizations and health care systems. Of particular note, the VA offers REACH VA as a routine program through its Program of General Caregiver Support Services (VA, 2020). REACH II and its adaptations have been administered by individuals from diverse professions, including nursing, social work, and counseling, in real-world care settings (Benjamin Rose Institute on Aging and FCA, 2020; Nichols et al., 2011). While the quantity and duration of in-home and telephone sessions vary among the different REACH II implementations, the authors of the REACH-TX adaptation note that the dose and intensity of the intervention can be gauged and modified through an initial risk assessment to evaluate personal and environmental challenges and needs for caregivers (Cho et al., 2019). They also explain that ongoing communications between the community organization and an evaluation team improved implementation and helped sustain a partnership with the intervention's funder. The authors state further that sustaining the intervention was possible through monetary and institutional support from the health care system, continuing education for health care providers, and incorporation of the intervention training into orientation for new nurses (Stevens et al., 2012).

Several challenges to implementing REACH II interventions were also uncovered across the various adaptations. In DE-REACH, just 70 percent of the basic modules described in the intervention manual could be executed (Berwig et al., 2017). Local funding for the community organization implementing REACH II (North Texas) was insufficient to support a comprehensive evaluation of the program (Lykens et al., 2014). A survey of organizations that have implemented REACH II or its adaptations found that the most frequent barriers to successful implementation were lack of internal organization resources, insufficient understanding of the program, and issues with participant enrollment and completion (Benjamin Rose Institute on Aging and FCA, 2020).

The authors of various REACH II adaptations have offered suggestions for future research that would help propel REACH II toward broad implementation and adoption. According to Cheung and colleagues (2014), an important step toward broad implementation would be pragmatic clinical trials. Similarly, Luchsinger and colleagues (2018) recommend modifying trial designs in future research on REACH II, conducting long-term studies that last more than 6 months, and including diverse sociodemographic groups in studies that are appropriately powered. Authors of two separate adaptations advocate for research on how modifying the intensity, dose, and duration of the intervention may impact its effectiveness (Berwig et al., 2017; Czaja et al., 2018).

Resources The total cost of the original REACH II intervention was $1,214 per caregiver, which included costs of staff training, staff labor for intervention delivery, caregiver time, travel expenses and travel time, and intervention materials (Nichols et al., 2008). The cost for a caregiver to gain an additional hour of time spent on noncaregiving activities was calculated as $4.96 per day for each caregiver enrolled in the program. Twelve months following the intervention, the persons living with dementia whose caregivers had been enrolled in REACH VA exhibited a cost savings (including drug costs) to the VA system of 25 percent compared with the control group and with 12 months prior to the intervention (Nichols et al., 2017). With implementation of REACH VA, the estimated average annual savings to the VA was predicted to be $4,338 per participant (Nichols et al., 2017).

Conclusion Regarding REACH II and Its Adaptations

As a whole, the evidence supporting REACH II and its adaptations is encouraging. Of particular note, REACH II has been studied in and adapted for diverse populations to a greater extent than is usual in the field. A moderate amount of evidence related to intervention acceptability, feasibility, and resource requirements is available.

CONCLUSION: REACH II and its adaptations—interventions that provide support for family care partners/caregivers through a combination of strategies that include problem solving, skills training, stress management, support groups, provision of information and education, and role playing—have demonstrated some effectiveness under clinical trial conditions and are already being implemented in a variety of community settings with promising results. These interventions are ready for the next stage of field testing to support their widespread adaptation to and adoption in a variety of settings where people seek dementia care. Those efforts will enhance understanding and information dissemination with respect to key factors in addition to effectiveness that are important for deciding whether and how to implement an intervention, such as determining the workforce and space needed; testing payment models and integration into workflow; and ensuring adaptations for different populations (e.g., racial/ethnic groups) and settings (e.g., rural areas).

Recommendations

Together, collaborative care models and REACH interventions are practical instantiations of many, but not all, core components of care, services, and supports that are important for persons living with dementia, care partners, and caregivers, as outlined in Chapter 2. These core components are detection and diagnosis; assessment of symptoms to inform planning and deliver care; information and education; medical management; support in activities of daily living; support for care partners and caregivers; communication and collaboration; coordination of medical care, long-term services and supports, and community-based services and supports; supportive and safe environment; and advance care planning and end-of-life care. These interventions also respond to priorities identified by persons living with dementia and their care partners and caregivers at the committee's public meetings, including the need for education, practical guidance, skills, and support, as well as challenges related to navigating a patchwork of often uncoordinated care systems, providers, and services.

The state of the evidence base for these two intervention types as assessed by the AHRQ review complicates making recommendations for a path forward. The AHRQ finding of low-strength evidence of effectiveness suggests limited confidence in the effectiveness of these interventions and indicates that additional evidence is likely to change the estimate of effect. Nevertheless, the committee recommends a path forward based on the following argument. First, given the inherent challenges of studying this topic—including the complexity of dementia care interventions, the diversity of populations affected, and the importance of contextual effects, as described in Chapter 3—the fact that these two interventions produced low-strength evidence of effectiveness is important. Second, there is a notable trend in benefits across multiple outcomes beyond those for which the AHRQ review was able to draw a conclusion, and the consistency of evidence of benefit across sources of evidence is encouraging. Third, there is a moderate amount of evidence to inform implementation as assessed against the EtD criteria. Particularly important, while more evidence is needed regarding the full range of populations that could benefit from these interventions, they have already been studied in diverse populations, although additional evidence is needed to expand understanding of their use in all populations.

Taken together, these considerations led the committee to conclude that the evidence is sufficient to justify implementation of these two types of interventions in a broad spectrum of community settings, with evaluation conducted to continue expanding the evidence base for future implementation. The committee believes that this approach to expanding the evidence base is likely to bring greater gains and better inform real-world implementation relative to focusing on additional large RCTs aimed at generating moderate- or high-strength evidence in a future systematic review before any further dissemination can be supported. These concepts are discussed in detail in the next chapter.

RECOMMENDATION 1: ***Implement and evaluate outcomes for collaborative care models in multiple and varied real-world settings under appropriate conditions for monitoring, quality improvement, and information sharing.***

To enhance the evidence base for decision making about the implementation of collaborative care models—which use multidisciplinary teams to integrate medical and psychosocial approaches to the care of persons living with dementia—agencies of the U.S. Department of Health and Human Services (HHS) should work with state Medicaid programs and health care systems to implement these interventions and evaluate their outcomes in multiple and varied real-world settings under appropriate conditions for monitoring, quality improvement, and information sharing. Along with adding to the current evidence for effectiveness, these efforts should include examining key factors that are important for determining whether and how to implement an intervention, such as identifying workforce and space needs, testing payment models and integration into workflow, and ensuring adaptations for different populations (e.g., racial/ethnic groups) and settings (e.g., rural areas). Specifically, to advance these efforts:

- **The Centers for Medicare & Medicaid Services should explore the value of collaborative care models offered as a benefit through Medicare Advantage programs and alternative payment models and for fee-for-service beneficiaries to build the infrastructure, train the workforce, and redesign the workflows that would facilitate the adoption, monitoring, and evaluation of these programs.**
- **State Medicaid programs serving persons living with dementia and dual-eligible beneficiaries should encourage participating health systems, systems that provide long-term services and supports, and managed care organizations to provide collaborative care for persons living with dementia. This care could be included in a dementia-focused quality metric.**
- **The National Institute on Aging, HHS's Office of the Assistant Secretary for Planning and Evaluation, the Agency for Healthcare Research and Quality, and the Administration for Community Living should support research and stakeholder engagement focused on collaborative care models to aid in scaling and sustaining the models; identifying monitoring and**

evaluation standards; developing monitoring and evaluation plans; and sharing information about key findings, lessons learned, and promising practices.

- Health care systems, including those in the U.S. Department of Veterans Affairs, should support infrastructure that would facilitate the collaboration of providers of primary care, mental health and other specialty care, and long-term services and supports within the health care system and with local home-based community services and supports agencies in implementing collaborative care models to improve the well-being of persons living with dementia and their care partners and caregivers.

RECOMMENDATION 2: *Implement and evaluate outcomes for REACH II and its adaptions in multiple and varied real-world settings under appropriate conditions for monitoring, quality improvement, and information sharing.*

To enhance the evidence base for decision making about the implementation of REACH II and its adaptations—a multicomponent intervention that provides support for family care partners and caregivers—agencies within the U.S. Department of Health and Human Services (HHS) should work with state agencies, community organizations, and care systems to implement and evaluate outcomes of these interventions in multiple and varied real-world settings under appropriate conditions for monitoring, quality improvement, and information sharing. Along with adding to the current evidence for effectiveness, these efforts should include examining key factors that are important for determining whether and how to implement an intervention, such as identifying workforce and space needs, testing payment models and integration into workflow, and ensuring adaptations for different populations (e.g., racial/ethnic groups) and settings (e.g., rural areas). Specifically, to advance these efforts:

- The Centers for Disease Control and Prevention and the Administration for Community Living should incorporate REACH II and its adaptations into its efforts to support evidence-based dementia programs at state and local public health departments in concert with community organizations.
- The Centers for Medicare & Medicaid Services should explore the value of REACH II and its adaptations offered as a benefit through Medicare Advantage programs and alternative payment models and for fee-for-service beneficiaries to build the infrastructure, train the workforce, and redesign the workflows

that would facilitate the adoption, monitoring, and evaluation of these programs.

- State Medicaid programs serving persons living with dementia and dual-eligible beneficiaries should encourage participating health systems, systems that provide long-term services and supports, and managed care organizations to provide REACH II and its adaptations for care partners and caregivers. This care could be included in a dementia focused quality metric.
- The National Institute on Aging, HHS's Office of the Assistant Secretary for Planning and Evaluation, the Agency for Healthcare Research and Quality, and the Administration for Community Living should support research and stakeholder engagement focused on REACH II and its adaptations to aid in scaling and sustaining the model; identifying monitoring and evaluation standards; developing monitoring and evaluation plans; and sharing information about key findings, lessons learned, and promising practices.
- The U.S. Department of Veterans Affairs should participate in monitoring, quality improvement, and information-sharing initiatives to enable other entities to learn from its implementation of this intervention.
- Health care systems should support infrastructure that would facilitate the collaboration of providers of primary care, mental health and other specialty care, and long-term services and supports within the health care system and with local home-based community services and supports agencies in implementing REACH II and its adaptations to improve the well-being of persons living with dementia and their care partners and caregivers.

It is important to stress that these recommendations should not be taken to imply that these are the only two types of interventions that should be pursued. As discussed next, additional research on a full range of interventions should be undertaken to continue to innovate and develop better ways of meeting the urgent needs of persons living with dementia, care partners, and caregivers.

IMPROVING AND EXPANDING THE EVIDENCE BASE FOR DEMENTIA CARE INTERVENTIONS: GAPS AND OPPORTUNITIES

For the majority of dementia care interventions included in the AHRQ systematic review, the evidence was insufficient to draw conclusions regarding their effect on outcomes for persons living with dementia and/or their care partners and caregivers. However, a finding of insufficient evidence does not mean that an intervention is ineffective or that it should not be implemented. Rather, such a finding simply reflects the high uncertainty resulting from the limitations of the evidence base and the approach used in the AHRQ systematic review to synthesize and assess the strength of the existing evidence to support conclusions on readiness for broad dissemination and implementation. As discussed in Chapter 4, different stakeholders may use different criteria to inform decisions on the implementation of dementia care interventions, and the AHRQ systematic review acknowledges that even low-strength evidence is a difficult bar to reach given the complexity of dementia care interventions and the settings and systems in which they are implemented (as discussed in Chapter 3). If the magnitude of the effect of an intervention is small, or moderate but only for a specific subpopulation, that effect will be more difficult to detect. Thus, it is possible, and in some cases likely, that a dementia care intervention with insufficient evidence to support a conclusion on effectiveness may be beneficial for some populations in certain circumstances. To guide research investments going forward and to extract the maximum value from the large body of interventions for which the AHRQ review found the evidence to be insufficient, the committee sought to identify gaps in and opportunities to improve and expand the evidence base for dementia care interventions.

This section first details the committee's approach to assessing the state of the evidence for dementia care interventions other than the two interventions discussed in the previous section—collaborative care models and REACH II and its adaptations—and identifying gaps in and opportunities for expanding and improving that evidence base. The sections that follow detail the findings of this assessment first for interventions targeting the community, policy, and societal levels and then for those targeting the individual level.

Approach to Assessing the State of the Evidence for Other Interventions and Identifying Gaps and Opportunities

Consistent with the study charge, the committee's approach to assessing the state of the evidence for interventions other than collaborative care models and REACH II and adaptations relied heavily on the findings from the AHRQ systematic review. However, the committee also considered additional sources of evidence, including expert and stakeholder input and such resources as Best Practice Caregiving, a database resulting from a joint project of the Benjamin Rose Institute on Aging, the Family Caregiver Alliance, and the Gerontological Society of America. Best Practice Caregiving provides information derived from real-world implementation of interventions (Benjamin Rose Institute on Aging and FCA, 2020) and was helpful in identifying interventions (or adaptations thereof) evaluated in the AHRQ systematic review that had been implemented in practice settings, although the committee did not systematically evaluate the evidence of effectiveness captured in the database.

The committee also mapped the interventions in the AHRQ systematic review against the framework for dementia care interventions presented in Chapter 3. This mapping exercise made it possible to assess the balance among interventions targeting the individual, community, policy, and societal levels, all of which are important to meeting the needs of persons living with dementia, care partners, and caregivers.

In addition, the committee sought to understand the degree to which the AHRQ review's findings of insufficient evidence resulted from a lack of evidence or from other limitations of the evidence base that prevented drawing conclusions about readiness for broad dissemination and implementation. Where evidence was lacking, the committee leveraged stakeholder input from its information-gathering process to identify opportunities for future research that would expand the evidence for interventions that have been identified by persons living with dementia, care partners, and caregivers as important to their health and well-being. (Opportunities to expand the evidence base for collaborative care models and multicomponent interventions such as REACH II that provide support to caregivers in a variety of ways are discussed in the preceding section.) For those categories of interventions (e.g., exercise, psychosocial interventions) for which the AHRQ review's analytic set[5] includes a multitude of RCTs and for which there was some signal of benefit and little or no evidence of harm, the committee identified important gaps that posed barriers to the synthesis and interpretation of the evidence. Signal of benefit was determined based on the observation of benefit for a given outcome in multiple independent RCTs evaluating the same (or a similar) intervention, even if the overall body of evidence was mixed for that outcome (i.e., one or more RCTs found no benefit for that outcome).[6] Although a signal of benefit may be insufficient to recommend interventions for broad dissemination and implementation—the focus of the AHRQ systematic review—this approach enabled the committee to

[5] As discussed previously, the AHRQ review excluded studies from the analytic set if they were judged to be pilot studies, had small sample sizes, or were rated as having high risk of bias.

[6] For the purposes of this assessment, benefit was defined based on statistical significance, consistent with the AHRQ systematic review. However, the committee recognizes that the ability to achieve statistical significance depends on the sample size and that failure to detect a statistically significant effect does not necessarily mean that an intervention failed to provide benefit for some people or in some circumstances. Trends in the primary data that show improvement over time (or with increased intervention intensity) may support conclusions regarding benefit even in the absence of statistical significance.

highlight opportunities to address gaps and advance evidence-based practice for dementia care.

Gaps and Opportunities for Interventions Targeting the Community, Policy, and Societal Levels

In addition to individual-level interventions, discussed in the next section, community-, policy-, and societal-level interventions have the potential to improve the health and well-being of persons living with dementia and their care partners and caregivers by changing the systems and settings in which they receive care, services, and supports (e.g., by targeting the organization, financing, and delivery processes). However, much of the focus on promising interventions in the field has been on those targeting individual persons living with dementia, care partners, and caregivers. The AHRQ systematic review and a recent Lancet Commission report (Livingston et al., 2020) used different approaches to evaluate the evidence, but both focused heavily on individual-level interventions, highlighting an evidence gap related to community-, policy-, and societal-level strategies.[7]

In addition to the collaborative care models described earlier in this chapter, other community-level interventions evaluated in the AHRQ systematic review included case management, implementation of care protocols (descriptions of procedures, processes, and tools for providing care in an organization or care delivery system), and care staff education and training. With the exception of collaborative care models, however, the AHRQ analytic set included few if any studies for most of these interventions. Moreover, all of these interventions target systems for the delivery of care, services, and supports. Completely absent from the AHRQ systematic review are policy- and societal-level interventions, such as dementia-friendly community initiatives and social insurance policies that would provide coverage for home- and community-based long-term care.

The paucity of evidence identified for interventions beyond the individual level in the AHRQ systematic review may be due in part to the challenges involved in studying these interventions. They often are not well suited to evaluation using the kinds of study designs that are likely to meet the evidence criteria used by AHRQ for its systematic reviews. Notably, the AHRQ review included no nonrandomized studies, but an RCT of

[7] Of note, the AHRQ systematic review refers to respite care and social support as programs delivered at the community and societal levels. While the availability of such programs may depend on community resources and policies, their implementation is at the individual level, and the committee therefore classifies them as individual-level interventions for the purposes of this report.

an intervention that increases paid leave for caregivers, for example, is unlikely to be feasible. Rather, evaluation methods such as those used for policy demonstration projects may be more appropriate for assessing the effectiveness of such policy interventions. As discussed further in Chapter 6, the committee urges that investment in future research on dementia care interventions include a focus on how better to study these kinds of interventions with rigor. Also vital is that evidence from studies not designed as RCTs be incorporated into future efforts to synthesize the evidence on dementia care interventions, even if there is a greater risk of bias related to the nonrandomized design. For example, one evidence synthesis methodology designed specifically to consider evidence on community-level interventions targeting population-level outcomes is that used by the Guide to Community Preventive Services (The Community Guide). Because RCTs are often difficult or inappropriate to conduct for public health interventions, The Community Guide does not privilege evidence from RCTs, but considers the suitability of the study design and the quality of execution for each quantitative study included in the body of evidence (Briss et al., 2000).

Additional challenges stem from the way interventions are defined and the consequences for search strategies used in the AHRQ systematic review. Policies and community-level programs and organizational structures may not be recognized as interventions per se. For example, the AHRQ review did not include studies on dementia villages—residential settings designed and operated around the care and support needs of persons living with dementia. At the committee's public workshop in April 2020, Mary Butler of the Minnesota Evidence-based Practice Center indicated that those studies had been excluded because they were considered to be evaluations of the effectiveness of care delivery settings rather than intervention studies.[8] The AHRQ systematic review notes that some community services and supports approaches, such as referral services and awareness-raising outreach, may have been missed because of the challenges of designing effective search strategies for such interventions in the context of a review with such broad scope. Going forward, adopting a broader definition of what constitutes a dementia care intervention may ensure that resources are invested in evaluating community-, policy-, and societal-level interventions and that such evaluations are included in future efforts to take stock of the state of the evidence.

> *CONCLUSION: The evidence base for dementia care interventions appears to be biased toward those targeting the individual*

---

[8] Presented by Mary Butler of the Minnesota Evidence-based Practice Center at the Care Interventions for Individuals with Dementia and Their Caregivers workshop on April 15, 2020.

level. The gap in the evidence for interventions targeting the community, policy, and societal levels may result from the way interventions are defined and the challenges of studying these kinds of interventions with rigor. Expanding the evidence base for such interventions will require investment in research that uses appropriate study designs, engages key stakeholders, and characterizes critical features of implementation. To support conclusions on the effectiveness of such interventions, synthesis methods will need to enable the evaluation of evidence on complex interventions derived from nonrandomized studies.

Gaps and Opportunities for Interventions Targeting the Individual Level

Although the evidence base for interventions targeting the individual level is larger as a whole relative to that for community-, policy-, and societal-level interventions, the AHRQ review determined that for all but collaborative care models and REACH II and its adaptations, the evidence was insufficient to draw conclusions regarding their effect on outcomes for persons living with dementia and/or their care partners and caregivers. The committee identified several gaps related to the quality and heterogeneity of the evidence for other individual-level interventions that need to be addressed to better support decision makers seeking guidance on which interventions are ready for broad dissemination and implementation. These gaps are described in the sections below, with interventions included in the AHRQ systematic review used to illustrate the issues involved and the opportunities to expand knowledge about what works, for whom, and in what conditions.

Gaps in High-Quality Evidence

For the majority of the individual-level interventions evaluated in the AHRQ systematic review, including some identified by persons living with dementia, care partners, and caregivers as important for their health and well-being, few if any studies met the criteria for inclusion in the analytic set, indicating a paucity of high-quality evidence to support conclusions regarding intervention effectiveness. As discussed previously, in many cases, studies captured through the AHRQ literature search were classified as small-scale and/or pilot studies or were assessed as having high risk of bias. While it is possible that inclusion of small trials and pilot studies could have bolstered the number of studies contributing evidence on effectiveness for some interventions, the systematic review team deemed them unsuitable for supporting conclusions on readiness for broad dissemination and implementation.

As discussed further in Chapter 6, future research can address these gaps by facilitating the evaluation of interventions through larger and longer-duration studies in real-world settings and using methodological approaches that decrease the potential for bias to reduce certainty in the findings of the study. As noted in the AHRQ systematic review, changes in research funding requirements in the past 5 years are already driving improvements in the methodological rigor of studies of dementia care interventions (Butler et al., 2020). Ongoing and future studies characterized by more stringent data monitoring and reporting, therefore, are likely to give rise to an evidence base that supports stronger conclusions regarding intervention effectiveness. The sections below highlight opportunities to expand and improve the evidence base for the following categories of interventions with the potential to make meaningful differences in the lives of persons living with dementia, care partners, and caregivers:

- late-stage care interventions,
- respite care,
- social support, and
- training and support for direct care workers.

Late-stage care interventions The importance of models of care that meet the needs of persons living with dementia and care partners/caregivers across the full continuum of dementia stages, including early- and late-stage care, has been recognized (Gitlin and Maslow, 2018). Interventions relevant to early-stage care (e.g., educational interventions) are discussed in other sections below; this section focuses specifically on those late-stage care interventions included in the AHRQ systematic review.

Late-stage care interventions encompass care, services, and supports designed to anticipate and meet the unique care needs of persons in the late stages of dementia and their caregivers. Late-stage care interventions evaluated in the AHRQ systematic review include decision aids and supportive interventions for decision making about feeding options, advance care planning, and palliative care (Butler et al., 2020). Decision aids, a set of evidence-based tools, can be used to guide caregivers in decision making regarding care for persons living with advanced dementia. For example, such decision aids may provide information about feeding options, including feeding tubes and assisted oral feeding, for persons living with dementia who are experiencing problems related to eating, such as difficulty swallowing (dysphagia). Decision aids may also be used to facilitate advance care planning, which can help reduce uncertainties about the wishes and goals of persons living with dementia as the disease progresses and may increase the incorporation of palliative care content into care plans (Livingston et al., 2020). The overarching aim of palliative care services is to reduce bothersome symptoms, distress, and hospitalization burden while increasing the comfort of persons living with dementia and their caregivers (Butler et al., 2020).

Participants in the 2017 National Research Summit on Care, Services, and Supports for Persons with Dementia and Their Caregivers emphasized the need for future such activities to focus specifically on care and services for late-stage dementia and end of life (Gitlin and Maslow, 2018). Included in one of the recommendations resulting from the 2017 summit was the need to identify effective approaches for helping persons living with dementia participate in their health care decisions, including person-centered advance care planning and end-of-life decisions. This recommendation is consistent with the tenets of supported decision making, which focuses on enabling people to make decisions about their own life and to be involved in decisions that affect their care (Donnelly, 2019).

Despite the importance ascribed to these issues, the AHRQ systematic review found little in the way of high-quality evidence to guide effective late-stage dementia care practices and advance supported decision making. The AHRQ review included one cluster RCT for an advance care planning intervention (a video for medical decision makers of persons living with dementia), but, compared with usual care, no benefit was observed for the outcome of burdensome treatments for persons living with dementia, such as hospital transfers or feeding tube insertions, or for the caregiver outcomes related to "do not hospitalize" directives, goals-of-care discussions, and decision makers' preference for comfort care (Mitchell et al., 2018). Another cluster RCT compared a print decision aid for feeding options with usual care and reported a benefit for persons living with dementia, as measured by the number of persons receiving a specialized dysphagia diet after 3 months (Hanson et al., 2011). Benefits were also reported for caregivers, as measured by a reduction in decisional conflict compared with the control group and an increase in the frequency of feeding discussions held with medical care providers. No studies on palliative care were included in the AHRQ analytic set, primarily because of high risk of bias.

Respite care Respite care interventions provide a means for care partners/caregivers to have temporary breaks from caregiving that may range from a few hours in a day to one or more full days (Butler et al., 2020). These interventions may include services through which in-home care is provided for persons living with dementia, adult day programs, and institutional respite services.

The AHRQ systematic review process identified three unique studies on respite care interventions (Lawton et al., 1989; Vandepitte et al., 2019; Zarit et al., 1998), but none were included in the analytic set because of high risk of bias. The paucity of evidence on respite care captured in the systematic review may have resulted in part from the challenges of evaluating such services through traditional RCTs (Zarit et al., 2017), and may be addressed through the application of methodologically robust nonrandomized study designs. Although the AHRQ systematic review found little evidence to support its effectiveness, respite care has been identified by caregivers as important for their well-being (Jennings et al., 2017).[9] At the committee's public meetings, persons living with dementia emphasized the need to address access issues related to personal expense for respite care (in-home and adult day programs),[10,11] suggesting the potential for policy interventions to improve the real-world effectiveness of respite care.

Social support Social support interventions, which may be delivered through in-person meetings, over the phone, or via web-based platforms (e.g., chat groups), are designed to provide care partners/caregivers with social interaction in addition to information and resources (Butler et al., 2020). Social support interventions, including peer support groups, were identified by caregivers as beneficial in their personal experience and deserving of priority attention in future research.[12,13] At the committee's April 2020 public workshop, Douglas Pace of the Alzheimer's Association discussed the results from 3,000 listening sessions with persons living with dementia and care partners/caregivers from across the organization's chapter network around the country, and noted that social support groups and the education they can provide were consistently identified as very important.[14] However, the AHRQ systematic review found little evidence to support conclusions on the effectiveness of these interventions. The analytic set included only two studies of these interventions: one RCT compared in-person, peer-led mutual support groups for caregivers with usual care (Wang et al., 2012), and another evaluated an automated phone support system for caregivers (Mahoney et al., 2001, 2003). Caregiver outcomes evaluated in the two studies differed, precluding the aggregation of results across studies. Beneficial effects of the in-person support groups were reported for caregiver distress and quality of life (Wang et al., 2012).

[9] Presented by Janet Michel at the Care Interventions for Individuals with Dementia and Their Caregivers workshop on April 15, 2020.

[10] Presented by Janet Michel at the Care Interventions for Individuals with Dementia and Their Caregivers workshop on April 15, 2020.

[11] Presented by Brian Van Buren at the Care Interventions for Individuals with Dementia and Their Caregivers public meeting on May 29, 2020.

[12] Presented by Brian Van Buren at the Care Interventions for Individuals with Dementia and Their Caregivers public meeting on May 29, 2020.

[13] Presented by Maria Martinez Israelite at the Care Interventions for Individuals with Dementia and Their Caregivers public meeting on May 29, 2020.

[14] Presented by Douglas Pace of the Alzheimer's Association at the Care Interventions for Individuals with Dementia and Their Caregivers workshop on April 15, 2020.

Training and support for direct care workers The AHRQ systematic review evaluated interventions targeting the well-being of direct care workers separately from those targeting the well-being of unpaid care partners and caregivers (Butler et al., 2020). Interventions for direct care workers were focused on reducing stress and burnout, for example, through peer support and training in stress management and relaxation techniques. The results from the systematic review indicate that the evidence base for such interventions is very preliminary, with only three small pilot studies being captured in the literature search (Barbosa et al., 2015; Davison et al., 2007; Visser et al., 2008), none of which was included in the analytic set.

> CONCLUSION: *While there have been important advances in knowledge regarding ways to better provide care, support, and services for persons living with dementia and their care partners and caregivers, significant gaps remain in the evidence base for many interventions evaluated in the AHRQ systematic review, including interventions identified by persons living with dementia, care partners, and caregivers as important to their health and well-being. To address these gaps, future research investments will need to ensure that studies are appropriately designed and conducted with methodological rigor, and progress beyond pilot and efficacy studies to include the evaluation of interventions in real-world settings.*

> CONCLUSION: *Direct care workers often play important roles in meeting the needs of persons living with dementia throughout the different stages of the disease. Despite the potential for such care providers to experience work-related stress and burnout, however, the vast majority of interventions targeting caregiver well-being were aimed at unpaid care partners and caregivers. The benefits of training and support for direct care workers are understudied and represent a notable gap that warrants emphasis in future research.*

Gaps Related to Heterogeneity and Complexity

For some interventions included in the AHRQ systematic review, the challenge related to a finding of insufficient evidence was not a lack of quality studies as much as the difficulty of synthesizing the evidence and drawing conclusions about effectiveness given the substantial heterogeneity in the sampled populations, intervention implementation (e.g., components, settings, other contextual factors), and measurement and reporting of outcomes. As a result of these challenges, discussed further in the paragraphs that follow, mixed results across studies are difficult to interpret. Consequently, despite the availability of evidence from multiple RCTs, little is known regarding for whom these interventions work and how they need to be implemented.

As noted in the AHRQ systematic review, the diverse etiology and progressive nature of dementia add complexity to the evaluation of care interventions. Given that the need for care, services, and supports and the settings in which they are delivered change over the course of the disease, interventions may be more or less effective for individuals at different stages of disease progression. Yet, participants in a given study may have dementia ranging from mild to severe, introducing the potential for variable effects that may mask the benefit of the intervention in a subgroup. Additional variability is introduced when synthesizing evidence across studies that enrolled participants in different stages of dementia. Moreover, results from some studies that conducted subgroup analyses suggest that the effects of interventions can differ across subpopulations with different types of dementia (Alzheimer's versus other dementias) (Toots et al., 2016).

It is also important to note the potential for variation in the experiences and circumstances of care partners and caregivers who may be targeted by interventions or involved in the delivery of interventions to those for whom they are providing care and/or support. For example, the needs and capabilities of first-time care partners or caregivers may differ from those of individuals who have previously served in these roles. In some cases, multiple care partners or caregivers may be sharing the responsibility for providing care for a person living with dementia, and in other cases, people with mild cognitive impairment or early-stage dementia may themselves be care partners or caregivers for someone experiencing a more advanced stage of the disease. Such variation in care partner and caregiver circumstances may have implications for the perceived value of interventions, the fidelity of implementation, and intervention effectiveness that need to be better understood.

Beyond the challenges related to heterogeneity in the circumstances (types and stages of dementia, caregiving situations) of those individuals enrolled in studies, the dearth of data for specific demographic subpopulations further hinders drawing conclusions about the real-world effectiveness of dementia care interventions. Important subpopulations to consider in the context of research on dementia care interventions include major racial/ethnic groups, LGBTQ populations, people with significant comorbidities (e.g., hearing loss or vision impairment), people of low socioeconomic status, and those who reside in low-resource areas (e.g., rural and tribal populations). In addition to variation in the efficacy of interventions across these groups, access to interventions and feasibility of implementation may vary as well. Thus, even for those interventions showing promise in clinical trials, the applicability of the evidence to the full range of populations experiencing dementia is unclear.

Given these challenges related to population heterogeneity, improved reporting of participant demographics and subgroup analyses may help ensure that future research is better able to support conclusions on which interventions are effective for whom and under what circumstances. However, there are also opportunities for future research to help elucidate how interventions may be tailored to better meet the needs of specific subpopulations with respect not only to cultural appropriateness but also to such factors as degree of dementia-related impairment. For example, care interventions designed primarily for an older population may need to be adapted for individuals with early-onset dementia. Similarly, interventions designed for implementation in the context of long-term care facilities may need to be adapted for community-dwelling individuals with early-stage dementia. Recruitment of the diverse populations an intervention purports to serve, along with improved reporting and subgroup analyses, can further strengthen the evidence used to make decisions regarding implementation.

For complex interventions such those evaluated in the AHRQ systematic review, grouping interventions for the purpose of synthesizing the evidence often requires some trade-off between ensuring a body of evidence of adequate size and introducing heterogeneity that can make interpretation of the findings difficult. The AHRQ review acknowledges this challenge, especially in the absence of a field-accepted taxonomy for classifying dementia care interventions (Butler et al., 2020). Given the scope of the review, the categories of interventions were necessarily broad, with, in some cases, substantial variability in the components of interventions and/or how they were implemented. Such variability can contribute to a lack of consistency in results across studies of interventions within a category, making it difficult to draw conclusions about intervention effectiveness. Added to these challenges was insufficient detail in studies' descriptions of interventions, which hinders determining the comparability of studies, assessing fidelity, and interpreting differences in findings across studies.

In contrast to studies of interventions aimed at the prevention or treatment of dementia, which generally focus on a limited number of clinical endpoints, care intervention studies cover a wide range of outcomes for both persons living with dementia and care partners/caregivers enrolled in the studies. These outcomes include (but are not limited to) depression; agitation; anxiety; daily function; neuropsychological symptoms; and even highly specific outcomes, such as hyperphagic (excessive eating) behavior. Adding to this complexity is the use of different scales to measure the same outcome, potentially resulting in discrepant results even within studies. For some interventions, moreover, process outcomes (such as discussions with clinical providers) may be reported in addition to outcomes related to health and well-being. This variability in reported outcomes hampers assessment of the consistency of findings across studies of similar interventions and precluded quantitative pooling of data and meta-analysis for most interventions included in the AHRQ review. Harmonization of outcomes may help address these challenges, but efforts to define core sets of outcomes will need to include a focus on those used to evaluate benefits and harms, with particular emphasis on endpoints important to persons living with dementia, care partners, and caregivers. As noted in the AHRQ systematic review, few studies have reported on harms and other unintended consequences or on some outcomes (personhood, identity, well-being) valued by persons living with dementia, care partners, and caregivers (Butler et al., 2020). Evaluation of such outcomes is difficult using quantitative metrics and may necessitate further investment in qualitative and mixed-method research designs.

The sections below highlight types of interventions that illustrate the challenges to evaluating dementia care interventions posed by the heterogeneity issues reviewed above, as well as the value of future research and evidence synthesis approaches aimed at elucidating the populations/settings for which interventions are effective and how they should be implemented to achieve outcomes that are important to persons living with dementia, care partners, and caregivers. The following categories of interventions are discussed:

- exercise,
- music,
- psychosocial interventions, and
- cognitive interventions.

Exercise Exercise and physical activity are important contributors to healthy aging, with benefits related to both physical and cognitive function (Livingston et al., 2020; NASEM, 2017). In discussions with the committee, persons living with dementia and care partners/caregivers indicated that exercise is an important part of staying active[15] and that physical activity helps with mental health and coping.[16]

Exercise was the intervention category with the second largest body of studies meeting the criteria for inclusion in the AHRQ systematic review; the analytic set included 10 studies, 3 of which were cluster RCTs (Butler et al., 2020). However, the implementation of exercise interventions and the outcomes evaluated varied across studies. Exercise interventions included aerobic, strength, or balance training, alone or in combination and with variable levels of intensity. Settings and formats (i.e., individual versus group) also varied. Most study participants had mild to moderate dementia (a mix of Alzheimer's, vascular, and mixed dementias).

---

[15] Presented by Janet Michel at the Care Interventions for Individuals with Dementia and Their Caregivers workshop on April 15, 2020.

[16] Presented by Maria Martinez Israelite at the Care Interventions for Individuals with Dementia and Their Caregivers public meeting on May 29, 2020.

Despite this heterogeneity, benefit was observed for several outcomes for persons living with dementia in more than one RCT, providing a signal of effectiveness. Of eight studies that evaluated the effect of exercise on daily function (Bossers et al., 2016; Chen et al., 2019; Hoffmann et al., 2016; Huang et al., 2019; Lamb et al., 2018; Pitkälä et al., 2013; Telenius et al., 2015; Toots et al., 2016), two reported beneficial effects of group exercise (Bossers et al., 2016; Pitkälä et al., 2013). Another study observed a positive effect of a hand exercise program on autonomous eating (Chen et al., 2019). Two studies reported on balance outcomes, both finding a benefit at one of two measured time points (Telenius et al., 2015; Toots et al., 2016). The effect of a high-intensity exercise on balance was greater for adults with non-Alzheimer's dementia than for those with Alzheimer's dementia (Toots et al., 2016). Of four exercise studies that measured the intervention effect on neuropsychiatric symptoms (Hoffmann et al., 2016; Huang et al., 2019; Lamb et al., 2018; Telenius et al., 2015), benefit was associated with group exercise in one study (Hoffmann et al., 2016) and with Tai Chi in another (Huang et al., 2019). In some cases, exercise was included as part of a multicomponent intervention. For example, group exercise is a core component of the Reducing Disabilities in Alzheimer's Disease (RDAD) multicomponent intervention, which has been shown to benefit persons living with dementia in the areas of health, depression, and function (days of restricted activity) (Teri et al., 2003). Given the broad benefits of physical activity and the lack of any clear link to serious adverse events (Butler et al., 2020), future research may be most impactful if focused on elucidating the optimal type, duration, format, and intensity of exercise interventions and the expected benefits at different stages of disease progression.

Music Music interventions are generally intended to be calming or pleasurable activities and may target cognitive and sensory stimulation. At the committee's public workshop, one caregiver described how enjoyment of music was an important aspect of quality of life for her and her husband, for whom she is providing care.[17] Another speaker noted that, despite the mixed research results, music has been helpful in practice for some people experiencing such feelings as loneliness and helplessness.[18]

The analytic set for the AHRQ systematic review included five RCTs of music interventions, but implementation and reported outcomes varied across studies, so that for most outcomes, assessment of strength of evi-

---

[17] Presented by Janet Michel at the Care Interventions for Individuals with Dementia and Their Caregivers workshop on April 15, 2020.

[18] Presented by Douglas Pace of the Alzheimer's Association at the Care Interventions for Individuals with Dementia and Their Caregivers workshop on April 15, 2020.

dence was based on a single RCT (Butler et al., 2020). The music interventions studied, which were often delivered in group settings, ranged from playing musical instruments to listening to recorded songs or singing and in some cases also involved body movement. The effect of music interventions on agitation in persons living with dementia was evaluated in three RCTs (Cheung et al., 2018; Lin et al., 2011; Sung et al., 2012), one of which reported benefit (Lin et al., 2011). Benefits were also observed for quality of life (Särkämö et al., 2013), mood (Särkämö et al., 2013), anxiety (Sung et al., 2012), and depression (Chu et al., 2014) in the single studies in which those outcomes were measured. In addition to the observed benefits for persons living with dementia, one study reported an improvement in family caregivers' burden associated with participation in a singing group (Särkämö et al., 2013). While these results provide some signal of benefit, future research may increase understanding of the comparative effectiveness of different types of music interventions for different populations and, given the variation in individual preferences, the importance of tailoring such interventions.

Psychosocial interventions The psychosocial intervention category within the AHRQ systematic review encompasses a diverse set of psychotherapeutic and psychoeducational interventions (Butler et al., 2020). The review classified psychosocial interventions based on whether they were targeted at addressing behavioral and psychological symptoms of dementia in persons living with dementia (e.g., through cognitive-behavioral training) or at improving the overall well-being of persons living with dementia or their care partners and caregivers (e.g., through skills training or counseling). Psychosocial interventions are generally delivered by highly trained health or social service professionals in one-on-one or group settings. In some cases, sessions involve dyads of persons living with dementia and care partners/caregivers. Although psychotherapeutic and psychoeducational interventions have distinct definitions, in practice they often share intervention components. As noted in the AHRQ systematic review, this makes it difficult to define subgroups of psychosocial therapies more narrowly for analysis at a more granular level. The resulting heterogeneity in interventions within this category poses a challenge for aggregating data and drawing conclusions about more specific interventions (or intervention components) that are effective.

The category of psychosocial therapies for care partner/caregiver well-being represented the largest body of included studies among the interventions evaluated in the AHRQ systematic review (29 studies) (Butler et al., 2020). Notably, however, the AHRQ analytic set included no studies of psychosocial therapies directly targeting persons living with dementia (for outcomes related to either behavioral and psychological symptoms of dementia [BPSD] or well-being). Benefits of psychosocial therapies for care partner/caregiver well-being were reported for multiple outcomes for both the caregivers to whom the interventions were targeted and the persons receiving care. While the results were mixed for all outcomes, this is not surprising given the variability in the interventions included in the category. For caregivers, psychosocial therapies were associated with benefits related to depression (in 8 of 12 studies measuring short-term outcomes and in 2 of 8 studies measuring long-term outcomes), burden (in 5 of 13 studies), bother/distress (in 4 of 9 studies), quality of life (in 6 of 14 studies), and caregiving confidence (in 3 of 6 studies). Approximately half of the studies included in the analytic set also reported on outcomes for persons living with dementia who were receiving care from those caregivers to whom the intervention was targeted. Benefits for persons living with dementia were observed for measures related to function (in 2 of 3 studies measuring short-term outcomes and in 1 of 5 studies measuring long-term outcomes), depression (in 2 of 5 studies), neuropsychiatric symptoms (in 3 of 6 studies measuring short-term outcomes but none of the 3 studies measuring long-term outcomes), quality of life (in 2 of 8 studies), institutionalization (in 1 of 4 studies), and health care usage (in 1 of 5 studies). It should also be noted that the majority of components in REACH II and its adaptations, described earlier in this chapter, map to the psychosocial intervention category.

During discussions with the committee, psychosocial therapies (e.g., counseling, education on both the disease and skills for caregivers) were identified as valued and beneficial interventions by both persons living with dementia[19,20,21] and care partners/caregivers.[22,23] In addition, the myriad psychotherapeutic and educational/skills-building interventions in the Best Practice Caregiving database (Benjamin Rose Institute on Aging and FCA, 2020) suggest that stakeholders operating in community-level practice-based settings see value in implementing these types of interventions.[24]

---

[19] Presented by Brian Van Buren at the Care Interventions for Individuals with Dementia and Their Caregivers public meeting on May 29, 2020.

[20] Presented by Cynthia Huling Hummel at the Care Interventions for Individuals with Dementia and Their Caregivers public meeting on May 29, 2020.

[21] Presented by John Richard (JR) Pagan at the Care Interventions for Individuals with Dementia and Their Caregivers public meeting on May 29, 2020.

[22] Presented by Janet Michel at the Care Interventions for Individuals with Dementia and Their Caregivers workshop on April 15, 2020.

[23] Presented by Maria Martinez Israelite at the Care Interventions for Individuals with Dementia and Their Caregivers public meeting on May 29, 2020.

[24] Of note, whether educational and skills-building interventions included in the Best Practice Caregiving database would have been classified as psychosocial or multicomponent interventions using the AHRQ systematic review taxonomy is often not clear because of the limitations of the intervention descriptions and the lack of consensus on taxonomies for dementia care interventions.

Monitoring and reporting of experiences with implementing different psychosocial interventions in these real-world settings, along with pragmatic research studies, may provide opportunities to elucidate the critical components of psychosocial interventions for persons living with dementia and care partners/caregivers. The evaluation of such interventions, however, would benefit from a clearer taxonomy.

Cognitive interventions The AHRQ systematic review evaluated several types of interventions targeting the cognitive function of persons living with dementia and/or their ability to carry out daily activities (Butler et al., 2020). These interventions included cognitive stimulation therapy, cognitive training, cognitive rehabilitation, and reminiscence therapy. While individual RCTs of such cognitive interventions suggest the potential for benefits ranging from improved quality of life (Orrell et al., 2014; Spector et al., 2003), to reduced depression (Li et al., 2019; Wang, 2007), to improvements in eating behavior (Hsu et al., 2017; Kao et al., 2016) in persons living with dementia, assessment of effectiveness was complicated by the lack of clear differentiation among the different intervention types. For example, cognitive training interventions aim to improve cognitive function (e.g., memory, reasoning, speed of processing) through repetitive or progressive drill-like exercises, while cognitive rehabilitation interventions similarly focus on cognitive abilities (such as memory and executive function) and may target the recovery or restoration of daily functions. Even within individual studies, terms for these two types of cognitive interventions are often used interchangeably. More consistent terminology and consensus on intervention taxonomies would aid in the comparison of interventions across studies and synthesis of the evidence to support conclusions on intervention effectiveness.

> CONCLUSION: *For some intervention categories, evidence is insufficient to support conclusions on readiness for broad dissemination and implementation, despite a multitude of RCTs providing some signal of benefit. As a result of heterogeneity in study populations, intervention implementation, and measured outcomes, little is known regarding which interventions are likely to be effective for persons living with dementia, care partners, and caregivers experiencing different stages of disease progression and how they should optimally be implemented.*

> CONCLUSION: *Evidence is lacking with respect to the effectiveness of dementia care interventions in diverse populations, such as specific racial/ethnic groups, LGBTQ populations, people with significant comorbidities or of low socioeconomic status, and those*

from low-resource areas (e.g., rural and tribal populations). Consequently, the applicability of the existing evidence base to the full range of persons living with dementia and their care partners and caregivers is not supported, even for those interventions showing promise in clinical trials.

Overarching Conclusion

CONCLUSION: The evidence needed to inform decisions about policy and the implementation of specific interventions broadly at the organizational and community levels—including informing the relative prioritization of many interventions that could be helpful but will require resources—is limited. Some challenges in the existing evidence base are due to the inherent complexity of the area of study, including the multifaceted nature of dementia, its heterogeneity across populations and settings, and its progression across different stages. However, the AHRQ systematic review also brings to the forefront some addressable limitations in the existing research base, such as a lack of diversity in study populations, underpowered and limited-duration studies, heterogeneity of outcome measures that precludes aggregation of results, lack of reporting on contextual factors that facilitate or impede intervention effectiveness, and research that is divorced from practical implementation needs.

REFERENCES

Alonso-Coello, P., H. J. Schünemann, J. Moberg, R. Brignardello-Petersen, E. A. Akl, M. Davoli, S. Treweek, R. A. Mustafa, G. Rada, S. Rosenbaum, A. Morelli, G. H. Guyatt, and A. D. Oxman. 2016. GRADE Evidence to Decision (EtD) frameworks: A systematic and transparent approach to making well informed healthcare choices. 1: Introduction. *BMJ* 353:i2016.

Amjad, H., S. K. Wong, D. L. Roth, J. Huang, A. Willink, B. S. Black, D. Johnston, P. V. Rabins, L. N. Gitlin, C. G. Lyketsos, and Q. M. Samus. 2018. Health services utilization in older adults with dementia receiving care coordination: The MIND at home trial. *Health Services Research* 53(1):556–579.

Archer, J., P. Bower, S. Gilbody, K. Lovell, D. Richards, L. Gask, C. Dickens, and P. Coventry. 2012. Collaborative care for depression and anxiety problems. *Cochrane Database of Systematic Reviews (Online)* 10.

Barbosa, A., M. Nolan, L. Sousa, A. Marques, and D. Figueiredo. 2015. Effects of a psychoeducational intervention for direct care workers caring for people with dementia: Results from a 6-month follow-up study. *American Journal of Alzheimer's Disease & Other Dementias* 31(2):144–155.

Bass, D. M., K. S. Judge, A. L. Snow, N. L. Wilson, R. Morgan, W. J. Looman, C. A. McCarthy, K. Maslow, J. A. Moye, R. Randazzo, M. Garcia-Maldonado, R. Elbein, G. Odenheimer, and M. E. Kunik. 2013. Caregiver outcomes of partners in dementia care: Effect of a care coordination program for veterans with dementia and their family members and friends. *Journal of the American Geriatrics Society* 61(8):1377–1386.

Bass, D. M., K. S. Judge, A. Snow, N. L. Wilson, R. O. Morgan, K. Maslow, R. Randazzo, J. A. Moye, G. L. Odenheimer, E. Archambault, R. Elbein, P. Pirraglia, T. A. Teasdale, C. A. McCarthy, W. J. Looman, and M. E. Kunik. 2014. A controlled trial of partners in dementia care: Veteran outcomes after six and twelve months. *Alzheimer's Research & Therapy* 6(1):9.

Bass, D. M., K. S. Judge, K. Maslow, N. L. Wilson, R. O. Morgan, C. A. McCarthy, W. J. Looman, A. L. Snow, and M. E. Kunik. 2015. Impact of the care coordination program "partners in dementia care" on veterans' hospital admissions and emergency department visits. *Alzheimer's & Dementia: Translational Research & Clinical Interventions* 1(1):13–22.

Bass, D. M., T. Hornick, M. Kunik, K. S. Judge, B. Primetica, K. Kearney, J. Rentsch, C. McCarthy, and J. Grim. 2019. Findings from a real-world translation study of the evidence-based "partners in dementia care." *Innovation in Aging* 3(3):igz031.

Belle, S. H., L. Burgio, R. Burns, D. Coon, S. J. Czaja, D. Gallagher-Thompson, L. N. Gitlin, J. Klinger, K. M. Koepke, C. C. Lee, J. Martindale-Adams, L. Nichols, R. Schulz, S. Stahl, A. Stevens, L. Winter, and S. Zhang. 2006. Enhancing the quality of life of dementia caregivers from different ethnic or racial groups: A randomized, controlled trial. *Annals of Internal Medicine* 145(10):727–738.

Benjamin Rose Institute on Aging and FCA (Family Caregiver Alliance). 2020. *Best practice caregiving*. https://bpc.caregiver.org/#searchPrograms (accessed August 12, 2020).

Berwig, M., S. Heinrich, J. Spahlholz, N. Hallensleben, E. Brähler, and H.-J. Gertz. 2017. Individualized support for informal caregivers of people with dementia—Effectiveness of the German adaptation of REACH II. *BMC Geriatrics* 17(1):286.

Bossers, W. J., L. H. van der Woude, F. Boersma, T. Hortobágyi, E. J. Scherder, and M. J. van Heuvelen. 2016. Comparison of effect of two exercise programs on activities of daily living in individuals with dementia: A 9-week randomized, controlled trial. *Journal of the American Geriatrics Society* 64(6):1258–1266.

Boustani, M., C. A. Alder, C. A. Solid, and D. Reuben. 2019. An alternative payment model to support widespread use of collaborative dementia care models. *Health Affairs* 38(1):54–59.

Briss, P. A., S. Zaza, M. Pappaioanou, J. Fielding, L. Wright-De Agüero, B. I. Truman, D. P. Hopkins, P. D. Mullen, R. S. Thompson, S. H. Woolf, V. G. Carande-Kulis, L. Anderson, A. R. Hinman, D. V. McQueen, S. M. Teutsch, and J. R. Harris. 2000. Developing an evidence-based guide to community preventive services—Methods. The task force on community preventive services. *American Journal of Preventive Medicine* 18(1 Suppl):35–43.

Brown, A. F., S. D. Vassar, K. I. Connor, and B. G. Vickrey. 2013. Collaborative care management reduces disparities in dementia care quality for caregivers with less education. *Journal of the American Geriatrics Society* 61(2):243–251.

Burgio, L. D., I. B. Collins, B. Schmid, T. Wharton, D. McCallum, and J. Decoster. 2009. Translating the REACH caregiver intervention for use by area agency on aging personnel: The REACH OUT program. *The Gerontologist* 49(1):103–116.

Butler, M., J. E. Gaugler, K. M. C. Talley, H. I. Abdi, P. J. Desai, S. Duval, M. L. Forte, V. A. Nelson, W. Ng, J. M. Ouellette, E. Ratner, J. Saha, T. Shippee, B. L. Wagner, T. J. Wilt, and L. Yeshi. 2020. Care interventions for people living with dementia and their caregivers. *Comparative Effectiveness Review No. 231*. Rockville, MD: Agency for Healthcare Research and Quality. doi: 10.23970/AHRQEPCCER231.

Callahan, C. M., M. A. Boustani, F. W. Unverzagt, M. G. Austrom, T. M. Damush, A. J. Perkins, B. A. Fultz, S. L. Hui, S. R. Counsell, and H. C. Hendrie. 2006. Effectiveness of collaborative care for older adults with Alzheimer disease in primary care: A randomized controlled trial. *Journal of the American Medical Association* 295(18):2148–2157.

Callahan, C. M., M. A. Boustani, M. Weiner, R. A. Beck, L. R. Livin, J. J. Kellams, D. R. Willis, and H. C. Hendrie. 2011. Implementing dementia care models in primary care settings: The aging brain care medical home. *Aging & Mental Health* 15(1):5–12.

Chen, L. L., H. Li, X. H. Chen, S. Jin, Q. H. Chen, M. R. Chen, and N. Li. 2019. Effects of hand exercise on eating action in patients with Alzheimer's disease. *American Journal of Alzheimer's Disease and Other Dementias* 34(1):57–62.

Cheung, K. S., B. H. Lau, P. W. Wong, A. Y. Leung, V. W. Lou, G. M. Chan, and R. Schulz. 2014. Multicomponent intervention on enhancing dementia caregiver well-being and reducing behavioral problems among Hong Kong Chinese: A translational study based on REACH II. *International Journal of Geriatric Psychiatry* 30(5):460–469.

Cheung, D. S. K., C. K. Y. Lai, F. K. Y. Wong, and M. C. P. Leung. 2018. The effects of the music-with-movement intervention on the cognitive functions of people with moderate dementia: A randomized controlled trial. *Aging & Mental Health* 22(3):306–315.

Chien, W. T., and Y. M. Lee. 2008. A disease management program for families of persons in Hong Kong with dementia. *Psychiatric Services* 59(4):433–436.

Cho, J., S. Luk-Jones, D. R. Smith, and A. B. Stevens. 2019. Evaluation of REACH-TX: A community-based approach to the REACH II intervention. *Innovation in Aging* 3(3):igz022.

Chodosh, J., B. A. Colaiaco, K. I. Connor, D. W. Cope, H. Liu, D. A. Ganz, M. J. Richman, D. L. Cherry, J. M. Blank, P. Carbone Rdel, S. M. Wolf, and B. G. Vickrey. 2015. Dementia care management in an underserved community: The comparative effectiveness of two different approaches. *Journal of Aging Health* 27(5):864–893.

Chu, H., C.-Y. Yang, Y. Lin, K.-L. Ou, T.-Y. Lee, A. P. O'Brien, and K.-R. Chou. 2014. The impact of group music therapy on depression and cognition in elderly persons with dementia: A randomized controlled study. *Biological Research for Nursing* 16(2):209–217.

Czaja, S. J., D. Loewenstein, R. Schulz, S. N. Nair, and D. Perdomo. 2013. A videophone psychosocial intervention for dementia caregivers. *The American Journal of Geriatric Psychiatry* 21(11):1071–1081.

Czaja, S. J., C. C. Lee, D. Perdomo, D. Loewenstein, M. Bravo, J. H. Moxley, and R. Schulz. 2018. Community REACH: An implementation of an evidence-based caregiver program. *Gerontologist* 58(2):e130–e137.

Davison, T. E., M. P. McCabe, S. Visser, C. Hudgson, G. Buchanan, and K. George. 2007. Controlled trial of dementia training with a peer support group for aged care staff. *International Journal of Geriatric Psychiatry* 22(9):868–873.

Dham, P., S. Colman, K. Saperson, C. McAiney, L. Lourenco, N. Kates, and T. K. Rajji. 2017. Collaborative care for psychiatric disorders in older adults: A systematic review. *Canadian Journal of Psychiatry* 62(11):761–771.

Donnelly, M. 2019. Deciding in dementia: The possibilities and limits of supported decision-making. *International Journal of Law and Psychiatry* 66:101466.

Duru, O. K., S. L. Ettner, S. D. Vassar, J. Chodosh, and B. G. Vickrey. 2009. Cost evaluation of a coordinated care management intervention for dementia. *American Journal of Managed Care* 15(8):521–528.

Eloniemi-Sulkava, U., M. Saarenheimo, M.-L. Laakkonen, M. Pietilä, N. Savikko, H. Kautiainen, R. S. Tilvis, and K. H. Pitkälä. 2009. Family care as collaboration: Effectiveness of a multicomponent support program for elderly couples with dementia. Randomized controlled intervention study. *Journal of the American Geriatrics Society* 57(12):2200–2208.

Gilman, B., D. Whicher, R. Brown, N. McCall, S. Dale, L. Felland, R. Schmitz, J. Schurrer, L. Vollmer Forrow, M. Flick, J. Dezron, and R. Lakhani. 2020. *Evaluation of the health care innovation awards, round 2: Final report*. Cambridge, MA: Mathematica.

Gitlin, L. N., and K. Maslow. 2018. *National research summit on care, services, and supports for persons with dementia and their caregivers: Report to the National Advisory Council on Alzheimer's Research, Care, and Services*. https://aspe.hhs.gov/system/files/pdf/259156/FinalReport.pdf (accessed September 1, 2020).

Hanson, L. C., T. S. Carey, A. J. Caprio, T. J. Lee, M. Ersek, J. Garrett, A. Jackman, R. Gilliam, K. Wessell, and S. L. Mitchell. 2011. Improving decision-making for feeding options in advanced dementia: A randomized, controlled trial. *Journal of the American Geriatrics Society* 59(11):2009–2016.

Heintz, H., P. Monette, G. Epstein-Lubow, L. Smith, S. Rowlett, and B. P. Forester. 2020. Emerging collaborative care models for dementia care in the primary care setting: A narrative review. *American Journal of Geriatric Psychiatry* 28(3):320–330.

Hoffmann, K., N. A. Sobol, K. S. Frederiksen, N. Beyer, A. Vogel, K. Vestergaard, H. Brændgaard, H. Gottrup, A. Lolk, L. Wermuth, S. Jacobsen, L. P. Laugesen, R. G. Gergelyffy, P. Høgh, E. Bjerregaard, B. B. Andersen, V. Siersma, P. Johannsen, C. W. Cotman, G. Waldemar, and S. G. Hasselbalch. 2016. Moderate-to-high intensity physical exercise in patients with Alzheimer's disease: A randomized controlled trial. *Journal of Alzheimer's Disease* 50(2):443–453.

Hsu, C.-N., L.-C. Lin, and S.-C. Wu. 2017. The effects of spaced retrieval training in improving hyperphagia of people living with dementia in residential settings. *Journal of Clinical Nursing* 26(19–20):3224–3231.

Huang, N., W. Li, X. Rong, M. Champ, L. Wei, M. Li, H. Mu, Y. Hu, Z. Ma, and J. Lyu. 2019. Effects of a modified Tai Chi program on older people with mild dementia: A randomized controlled trial. *Journal of Alzheimer's Disease* 72:947–956.

Jennings, L. A., A. Palimaru, M. G. Corona, X. E. Cagigas, K. D. Ramirez, T. Zhao, R. D. Hays, N. S. Wenger, and D. B. Reuben. 2017. Patient and caregiver goals for dementia care. *Quality of Life Research* 26(3):685–693.

Jennings, L. A., S. Hollands, E. Keeler, N. S. Wenger, and D. B. Reuben. 2020. The effects of dementia care co-management on acute care, hospice, and long-term care utilization. *Journal of the American Geriatrics Society* 68(11):2500–2507.

Judge, K. S., D. M. Bass, A. L. Snow, N. L. Wilson, R. Morgan, W. J. Looman, C. McCarthy, and M. E. Kunik. 2011. Partners in dementia care: A care coordination intervention for individuals with dementia and their family caregivers. *Gerontologist* 51(2):261–272.

Kao, C.-C., L.-C. Lin, S.-C. Wu, K.-N. Lin, and C.-K. Liu. 2016. Effectiveness of different memory training programs on improving hyperphagic behaviors of residents with dementia: A longitudinal single-blind study. *Clinical Interventions in Aging* 11:707–720.

LaMantia, M. A., C. A. Alder, C. M. Callahan, S. Gao, D. D. French, M. G. Austrom, K. Boustany, L. Livin, B. Bynagari, and M. A. Boustani. 2015. The aging brain care medical home: Preliminary data. *Journal of the American Geriatrics Society* 63(6):1209–1213.

Lamb, S. E., B. Sheehan, N. Atherton, V. Nichols, H. Collins, D. Mistry, S. Dosanjh, A. M. Slowther, I. Khan, S. Petrou, and R. Lall. 2018. Dementia and physical activity (DAPA) trial of moderate to high intensity exercise training for people with dementia: Randomised controlled trial. *BMJ* 361:k1675.

Lawton, M. P., E. M. Brody, A. Saperstein, and M. Grimes. 1989. Respite services for caregivers: Research findings for service planning. *Home Health Care Services Quarterly* 10(1–2):5–32.

Lee, C. C., S. J. Czaja, and R. Schulz. 2010. The moderating influence of demographic characteristics, social support, and religious coping on the effectiveness of a multicomponent psychosocial caregiver intervention in three racial ethnic groups. *The Journal of Gerontology, Series B, Psychological Sciences and Social Sciences* 65b(2):185–194.

Li, M., J.-h. Lyu, Y. Zhang, M.-l. Gao, R. Li, P.-x. Mao, W.-j. Li, and X. Ma. 2019. Efficacy of group reminiscence therapy on cognition, depression, neuropsychiatric symptoms, and activities of daily living for patients with Alzheimer disease. *Journal of Geriatric Psychiatry and Neurology* 33(5):272–281.

Lin, Y., H. Chu, C.-Y. Yang, C.-H. Chen, S.-G. Chen, H.-J. Chang, C.-J. Hsieh, and K.-R. Chou. 2011. Effectiveness of group music intervention against agitated behavior in elderly persons with dementia. *International Journal of Geriatric Psychiatry* 26(7):670–678.

Livingston, G., J. Huntley, A. Sommerlad, D. Ames, C. Ballard, S. Banerjee, C. Brayne, A. Burns, J. Cohen-Mansfield, C. Cooper, S. G. Costafreda, A. Dias, N. Fox, L. N. Gitlin, R. Howard, H. C. Kales, M. Kivimäki, E. B. Larson, A. Ogunniyi, V. Orgeta, K. Ritchie, K. Rockwood, E. L. Sampson, Q. Samus, L. S. Schneider, G. Selbæk, L. Teri, and N. Mukadam. 2020. Dementia prevention, intervention, and care: 2020 report of the Lancet Commission. *The Lancet* 396(10248):413–446.

Luchsinger, J. A., L. Burgio, M. Mittelman, I. Dunner, J. A. Levine, C. Hoyos, D. Tipiani, Y. Henriquez, J. Kong, S. Silver, M. Ramirez, and J. A. Teresi. 2018. Comparative effectiveness of 2 interventions for Hispanic caregivers of persons with dementia. *Journal of the American Geriatrics Society* 66(9):1708–1715.

Lykens, K., N. Moayad, S. Biswas, C. Reyes-Ortiz, and K. P. Singh. 2014. Impact of a community based implementation of REACH II program for caregivers of Alzheimer's patients. *PLoS One* 9(2):e89290.

Mahoney, D. M., B. Tarlow, R. N. Jones, S. Tennstedt, and L. Kasten. 2001. Factors affecting the use of a telephone-based intervention for caregivers of people with Alzheimer's disease. *Journal of Telemedicine and Telecare* 7(3):139–148.

Mahoney, D. F., B. J. Tarlow, and R. N. Jones. 2003. Effects of an automated telephone support system on caregiver burden and anxiety: Findings from the REACH for TLC intervention study. *Gerontologist* 43(4):556–567.

Mitchell, S. L., M. L. Shaffer, S. Cohen, L. C. Hanson, D. Habtemariam, and A. E. Volandes. 2018. An advance care planning video decision support tool for nursing home residents with advanced dementia: A cluster randomized clinical trial. *JAMA Internal Medicine* 178(7):961–969.

Moberg, J., A. D. Oxman, S. Rosenbaum, H. J. Schünemann, G. Guyatt, S. Flottorp, C. Glenton, S. Lewin, A. Morelli, G. Rada, P. Alonso-Coello, E. Akl, M. Gulmezoglu, R. A. Mustafa, J. Singh, E. von Elm, J. Vogel, and J. Watine. 2018. The GRADE Evidence to Decision (EtD) framework for health system and public health decisions. *Health Research Policy and Systems* 16(1):45.

Morgan, R. O., D. M. Bass, K. S. Judge, C. F. Liu, N. Wilson, A. L. Snow, P. Pirraglia, M. Garcia-Maldonado, P. Raia, N. N. Fouladi, and M. E. Kunik. 2015. A break-even analysis for dementia care collaboration: Partners in dementia care. *Journal of Genernal Internal Medicine* 30(6):804–809.

NASEM (National Academies of Sciences, Engineering, and Medicine). 2017. *Preventing cognitive decline and dementia: A way forward*. Washington, DC: The National Academies Press.

NASEM. 2020. *Evidence-based practice for public health emergency preparedness and response*. Washington, DC: The National Academies Press.

Nichols, L. O., C. Chang, A. Lummus, R. Burns, J. Martindale-Adams, M. J. Graney, D. W. Coon, S. Czaja, and Resources for Enhancing Alzheimer's Caregivers Health II Investigators. 2008. The cost-effectiveness of a behavior intervention with caregivers of patients with Alzheimer's disease. *Journal of the American Geriatrics Society* 56(3):413–420.

Nichols, L. O., J. Martindale-Adams, R. Burns, M. J. Graney, and J. Zuber. 2011. Translation of a dementia caregiver support program in a health care system—REACH VA. *Archives of Internal Medicine* 171(4):353–359.

Nichols, L. O., J. Martindale-Adams, C. W. Zhu, E. K. Kaplan, J. K. Zuber, and T. M. Waters. 2017. Impact of the REACH II and REACH VA dementia caregiver interventions on healthcare costs. *Journal of the American Geriatrics Society* 65(5):931–936.

NORC at the University of Chicago. 2016. *Third annual report: HCIA disease-specific evaluation.* Bethesda, MD: NORC at the University of Chicago.

Orrell, M., E. Aguirre, A. Spector, Z. Hoare, R. T. Woods, A. Streater, H. Donovan, J. Hoe, M. Knapp, C. Whitaker, and I. Russell. 2014. Maintenance cognitive stimulation therapy for dementia: Single-blind, multicentre, pragmatic randomised controlled trial. *British Journal of Psychiatry* 204(6):454–461.

Pew Research Center. 2019a. *Internet/broadband fact sheet.* https://www.pewresearch.org/internet/fact-sheet/internet-broadband (accessed September 4, 2020).

Pew Research Center. 2019b. *Mobile fact sheet.* https://www.pewresearch.org/internet/fact-sheet/mobile/#mobile-phone-ownership-over-time (accessed September 3, 2020).

Pitkälä, K. H., M. M. Pöysti, M.-L. Laakkonen, R. S. Tilvis, N. Savikko, H. Kautiainen, and T. E. Strandberg. 2013. Effects of the Finnish Alzheimer disease exercise trial (FINALEX): A randomized controlled trial. *JAMA Internal Medicine* 173(10):894–901.

Possin, K. L., J. J. Merrilees, S. Dulaney, S. J. Bonasera, W. Chiong, K. Lee, S. M. Hooper, I. E. Allen, T. Braley, A. Bernstein, T. D. Rosa, K. Harrison, H. Begert-Hellings, J. Kornak, J. G. Kahn, G. Naasan, S. Lanata, A. M. Clark, A. Chodos, R. Gearhart, C. Ritchie, and B. L. Miller. 2019. Effect of collaborative dementia care via telephone and Internet on quality of life, caregiver well-being, and health care use: The care ecosystem randomized clinical trial. *JAMA Internal Medicine* 179(12):1658–1667.

Rosa, T. D., K. L. Possin, A. Bernstein, J. Merrilees, S. Dulaney, J. Matuoka, K. P. Lee, W. Chiong, S. J. Bonasera, K. L. Harrison, and J. G. Kahn. 2019. Variations in costs of a collaborative care model for dementia. *Journal of the American Geriatrics Society* 67(12):2628–2633.

Samus, Q. M., D. Johnston, B. S. Black, E. Hess, C. Lyman, A. Vavilikolanu, J. Pollutra, J. M. Leoutsakos, L. N. Gitlin, P. V. Rabins, and C. G. Lyketsos. 2014. A multidimensional home-based care coordination intervention for elders with memory disorders: The Maximizing Independence at Home (MIND) pilot randomized trial. *American Journal of Geriatric Psychiatry* 22(4):398–414.

Särkämö, T., M. Tervaniemi, S. Laitinen, A. Numminen, M. Kurki, J. K. Johnson, and P. Rantanen. 2013. Cognitive, emotional, and social benefits of regular musical activities in early dementia: Randomized controlled study. *Gerontologist* 54(4):634–650.

Shrestha, S., K. S. Judge, N. L. Wilson, J. A. Moye, A. L. Snow, and M. E. Kunik. 2011. Utilization of legal and financial services of partners in dementia care study. *American Journal of Alzheimer's Disease and Other Dementias* 26(2):115–120.

Spector, A., L. Thorgrimsen, B. Woods, L. Royan, S. Davies, M. Butterworth, and M. Orrell. 2003. Efficacy of an evidence-based cognitive stimulation therapy programme for people with dementia: Randomised controlled trial. *The British Journal of Psychiatry* 183:248–254.

Stevens, A. B., E. R. Smith, L. R. Trickett, and R. McGhee. 2012. Implementing an evidence-based caregiver intervention within an integrated healthcare system. *Translational Behavioral Medicine* 2(2):218–227.

Sung, H.-c., W.-l. Lee, T.-l. Li, and R. Watson. 2012. A group music intervention using percussion instruments with familiar music to reduce anxiety and agitation of institutionalized older adults with dementia. *International Journal of Geriatric Psychiatry* 27(6):621–627.

Telenius, E. W., K. Engedal, and A. Bergland. 2015. Long-term effects of a 12 weeks high-intensity functional exercise program on physical function and mental health in nursing home residents with dementia: A single blinded randomized controlled trial. *BMC Geriatrics* 15(1):158.

Teri, L., L. E. Gibbons, S. M. McCurry, R. G. Logsdon, D. M. Buchner, W. E. Barlow, W. A. Kukull, A. Z. LaCroix, W. McCormick, and E. B. Larson. 2003. Exercise plus behavioral management in patients with Alzheimer disease: A randomized controlled trial. *Journal of the American Medical Association* 290(15):2015–2022.

Thyrian, J. R., J. Hertel, D. Wucherer, T. Eichler, B. Michalowsky, A. Dreier-Wolfgramm, I. Zwingmann, I. Kilimann, S. Teipel, and W. Hoffmann. 2017. Effectiveness and safety of dementia care management in primary care: A randomized clinical trial. *JAMA Psychiatry* 74(10):996–1004.

Toots, A., H. Littbrand, N. Lindelöf, R. Wiklund, H. Holmberg, P. Nordström, L. Lundin-Olsson, Y. Gustafson, and E. Rosendahl. 2016. Effects of a high-intensity functional exercise program on dependence in activities of daily living and balance in older adults with dementia. *Journal of the American Geriatrics Society* 64(1):55–64.

VA (U.S. Department of Veterans Affairs). 2020. *Program of general caregiver support services (PGCSS).* https://www.caregiver.va.gov/Care_Caregivers.asp (accessed September 29, 2020).

Vandepitte, S., K. Putman, N. Van Den Noortgate, S. Verhaeghe, and L. Annemans. 2019. Effectiveness of an in-home respite care program to support informal dementia caregivers: A comparative study. *International Journal of Geriatric Psychiatry* 34(10):1534–1544.

Vickrey, B. G., B. S. Mittman, K. I. Connor, M. L. Pearson, R. D. Della Penna, T. G. Ganiats, R. W. Demonte, Jr., J. Chodosh, X. Cui, S. Vassar, N. Duan, and M. Lee. 2006. The effect of a disease management intervention on quality and outcomes of dementia care: A randomized, controlled trial. *Annals of Internal Medicine* 145(10):713–726.

Vilagut, G., C. G. Forero, A. Pinto-Meza, J. M. Haro, R. de Graaf, R. Bruffaerts, V. Kovess, G. de Girolamo, H. Matschinger, M. Ferrer, and J. Alonso. 2013. The mental component of the short-form 12 health survey (SF-12) as a measure of depressive disorders in the general population: Results with three alternative scoring methods. *Value in Health* 16(4):564–573.

Visser, S. M., M. P. McCabe, C. Hudgson, G. Buchanan, T. E. Davison, and K. George. 2008. Managing behavioural symptoms of dementia: Effectiveness of staff education and peer support. *Aging & Mental Health* 12(1):47–55.

Wang, J. J. 2007. Group reminiscence therapy for cognitive and affective function of demented elderly in Taiwan. *International Journal of Geriatric Psychiatry* 22(12):1235–1240.

Wang, L. Q., W. T. Chien, and I. Y. Lee. 2012. An experimental study on the effectiveness of a mutual support group for family caregivers of a relative with dementia in mainland China. *Contemporary Nurse* 40(2):210–224.

Zarit, S. H., M. A. Stephens, A. Townsend, and R. Greene. 1998. Stress reduction for family caregivers: Effects of adult day care use. *Journal of Gerontology, Series B, Psychological Sciences and Social Sciences* 53(5):S267–S277.

Zarit, S. H., L. R. Bangerter, Y. Liu, and M. J. Rovine. 2017. Exploring the benefits of respite services to family caregivers: Methodological issues and current findings. *Aging and Mental Health* 21(3):224–231.

6

A BLUEPRINT FOR FUTURE RESEARCH

Research on interventions for persons living with dementia and their care partners and caregivers has expanded greatly in the past three decades, with a better understanding of guiding principles and core components of dementia care, services, and supports (see Chapter 2). However, the findings of low-strength evidence in the Agency for Healthcare Research and Quality (AHRQ) systematic review highlight the need for a more rigorous and robust evidence base to inform decision making in this complex system. The evidence is lacking as a result of methodological challenges (see Chapter 5), inattention to all the key factors that go into implementation decision making (see Chapter 4), and the need for more ways to study this topic in the face of complexity (see Chapters 3 and 5). There are also key gaps in the evidence base for certain types of interventions, including at the community, policy, and societal levels (see Chapter 5).

In this chapter, the committee lays out a blueprint for future research on dementia care interventions by outlining the methodological improvements needed across the research enterprise to strengthen the evidence base at multiple levels, including prioritizing inclusive research and incorporating throughout the study process the priorities of persons living with dementia and their care partners and caregivers. Recognizing the complexity of dementia care interventions and the systems in which they operate, this chapter highlights the importance of partnerships to delivering care and implementing interventions, as well as the integration of multiple methodological approaches to provide a richer evidence base that accounts for this complexity. In addition, key factors for assessing the real-world effectiveness of dementia care interventions are presented at the end of the chapter, along with strategies for improving the assessment of individual-level interventions and expanding the focus on community-, policy-, and societal-level interventions.

METHODOLOGICAL IMPROVEMENTS

The AHRQ systematic review identified two types of interventions—collaborative care models and a multicomponent intervention for informal caregivers (REACH [Resources for Enhancing Alzheimer's Caregiver Health] II and its adaptations)—as supported by low-strength evidence of effectiveness. The evidence for all other interventions examined in the AHRQ systematic review was insufficient to support conclusions regarding effectiveness. Although the inherent complexity of the area of study (e.g., the multifaceted and progressive nature of dementia and heterogeneity across populations and settings) poses its own challenges to the generation of a robust evidence base for dementia care interventions, the AHRQ review also noted challenges related to methodological limitations, as discussed in Chapter 5 and described in more detail below (Butler et al., 2020). These limitations include small sample sizes and limited-duration studies; heterogeneity of outcome measures and interventions that precludes aggregation of study results; the lack of measures related to intended and unintended benefits and harms important to persons living with dementia, care partners, and caregivers; overreliance on randomized studies with insufficient integration of other relevant evidence; insufficient reporting in the field in terms of fidelity, detailed methodology (e.g., nature and dose of intervention components), and null findings or negative results; and a lack of focus on community-, policy- and societal-level interventions. Despite encompassing a large number of studies, the AHRQ review also cast a relatively narrow net in excluding certain larger pilot studies and observational analyses of programs and policies that may yield benefit. The AHRQ review was limited in its ability to draw conclusions for specific interventions because of the high level of uncertainty of the evidence (Butler et al., 2020). This section of the chapter presents the committee's recommendations for improving the evidence base across the field, with a focus on the addressable methodological limitations highlighted in Chapter 5.

Ensure a Balanced Portfolio of Short- and Longer-Term Studies with Sufficient Sample Sizes

Much of the dementia care research conducted to date has consisted of studies with small sample sizes and limited duration, making it challenging to detect significant effects. This limitation of the evidence base was highlighted in the AHRQ systematic review, in which the vast majority of studies had small samples (defined in the systematic review as fewer than 10 participants per study arm) or were pilots (generally considered as a small-scale test of the feasibility of delivering the intervention, although as discussed in Chapter 5, this category as implemented in the AHRQ systematic review encompassed a heterogeneous set of studies). These studies were included in the review's evidence map describing the overall landscape of evidence but were excluded from the analytic set, and the systematic review found insufficient evidence to support conclusions about effectiveness (Butler et al., 2020). Studies with small sample sizes have an important role in moving the field forward by enabling early testing and refinement of newly created interventions, as well as early feasibility and pilot testing, as described in Stage I of the National Institutes of Health (NIH) Stage Model for Behavioral Intervention Development (discussed in Chapter 4) (NIA, 2018). However, it is important that interventions ultimately advance through later stages of the NIH model to include efficacy testing, effectiveness research in diverse populations and settings, and dissemination and implementation. Given the heterogeneity of persons living with dementia, care partners, and caregivers, studies with larger sample sizes are needed to provide adequate power for detecting meaningful and statistically significant effects across subgroups (HHS, 2018).

In addition to sample size, the duration of a study is important to understanding the intervention effects on outcomes for persons living with dementia and their care partners and caregivers, and whether the intervention has been implemented successfully with sustainability and long-term fidelity. Recognizing the long trajectories of dementia and how the disease course unfolds over a decade or more, it may be appropriate to extend the observation period for some studies based on the study population (e.g., age and stage of disease among study participants) and expected outcomes. Longitudinal studies in community populations that are representative of persons living with dementia, care partners, and caregivers—as opposed to convenience samples often drawn from specialized clinics—may shed light on the progressive nature of the disease and how care, support, and service needs evolve. It will be important to understand whether an intervention implemented over the long term can adapt effectively to the changing needs of persons living with dementia, care partners, and caregivers, including the settings in which care is delivered (e.g., individual home, residential care facility, nursing home). It is also possible that certain interventions are effective at one phase of the disease and not others. Community-, policy-, and societal-level interventions are well aligned with study designs that extend over longer observation periods and larger populations in real-world settings (discussed further later in this chapter). In some cases, it may be desirable for persons living with dementia, care partners, and caregivers to adhere to an intervention indefinitely (e.g., interventions, such as physical activity, aimed at establishing healthy lifestyles). In such instances, it would be important to assess long-term outcomes and any mediating effects that might contribute to the observed effect (Emsley et al., 2009; Richiardi et al., 2013).

Longer-duration studies may be feasible with alternative funding approaches that would enable investigators to design trials that could be renewed after the typical initial National Institute on Aging (NIA) 3- to 5-year funding term. Such studies would also be facilitated by NIA's use of existing mechanisms and criteria that guide study sections in assessing initial proposals and renewal applications, including consideration of ways to overcome some of the research and methodological barriers specific to dementia care research that make the traditional pathways inhospitable to this type of research, or that are too focused on clinical trials. NIA might also consider providing a road map for researchers offering funding support for each stage of the NIH Stage Model, tailored to the unique challenges inherent in dementia care research. Particularly for longer-duration studies, methods need to be in place for addressing issues related to attrition and how best to retain study participants. While the inclusion criteria of the AHRQ systematic review did not impose a minimum duration or follow-up period, attrition bias was assessed differently if the duration of a study was less or more than 12 weeks (Butler et al., 2020). The review authors note that they allowed attrition to reach relatively high levels before assigning high risk of bias, an approach that is particularly important given the high likelihood of attrition due to death in longer-term studies in an elderly population. In addition, methods are needed for addressing issues related to blinding and preventing drift in how an intervention is implemented across the study and control groups.

To generate the robust evidence needed to move the field forward most efficiently, it will be important to have a balanced portfolio for dementia care research comprising short- and longer-term studies, all with sufficient sample sizes, including studies along the NIH Stage Model. As in other therapeutic areas (e.g., cancer, cardiovascular disease), development of this portfolio may include a strategic system for harvesting data from different types of studies (e.g., pilot, longitudinal, observational and quasi-experimental studies, and randomized controlled trials [RCTs]).

Use a Harmonized Core of Outcomes and a Taxonomy of Interventions to Enable Pooling of Study Findings

The variability of outcomes and measures used in dementia care research makes it challenging to pool results across studies for statistical analysis. Throughout the AHRQ systematic review, outcomes were often synthesized qualitatively for this reason (Butler et al., 2020). The problem is compounded by the difficulty of measuring social aspects of dementia (e.g., identity, autonomy, privacy, safety) and by the lack of sufficient measures that take into account how outcomes for persons living with dementia, care partners, and caregivers change in concert with the trajectory of illness, the helping network, and the environmental/service delivery context. Chapter 3 highlights this point, noting that outcomes related to quality of life and meaning are difficult to capture for persons living with dementia because of the cognitive impairments they experience, as well as the inherent goals of dementia care, services, and supports aimed at helping a person live well in the world. The AHRQ systematic review found that quality of life was rarely the outcome of primary interest in a study, and often not measured at all, despite its being a central goal of dementia care interventions (Butler et al., 2020). This gap may be due in part to the potential challenges of measuring quality of life as the disease progresses in persons living with dementia; however, a number of measures designed to assess this outcome in persons with late-stage Alzheimer's disease and other dementias are available (e.g., Weiner et al., 2000).

As noted in Chapter 5, the AHRQ systematic review also noted a lack of clarity in how individual interventions are described within specific intervention categories, with outcomes often being measured and reported inconsistently, making it challenging to assess the evidence base (Butler et al., 2020). Many research publications examined in this and other related systematic reviews use inconsistent terminology to describe a particular intervention, and such inconsistency can often lead to discrepancies in classification (Gaugler et al., 2017). For example, the AHRQ systematic review notes that the terms "cognitive rehabilitation" and "cognitive training" were used interchangeably to describe intervention components within a single article, although the two terms have different meanings and interpretations (Butler et al., 2020).

To address these limitations, the committee agrees with the recommendation of the AHRQ systematic review regarding the need for better and consistent measures and measurements of psychosocial outcomes in persons living with dementia (Butler et al., 2020). In particular, having a general measure of well-being that could be adopted broadly is critical, particularly given the lack of consensus in the field as to what outcomes are most important to measure and matter to stakeholders (discussed further below). A harmonized core of meaningful outcomes is also important to help research converge with practice and policy; for example, greater attention is needed to identifying the types of measures that align with the Centers for Medicare & Medicaid Services' (CMS's) coverage decisions. Relatedly, measures are needed to examine the economic impacts of an intervention on persons living with dementia, care partners and caregivers, and other stakeholders, including cost-effectiveness and long-term viability (e.g., Gitlin et al., 2010; Livingston et al., 2020b). Interventions that do not improve outcomes and reduce health care costs or provide enough benefit to justify additional expenditures are unlikely to be adopted beyond the research setting. Health care utilization and costs have implications for outcomes of importance to persons living with dementia, care partners, and caregivers, as well as the practicality of intervention dissemination (discussed further below).

In addition, a taxonomy of dementia care interventions needs to be developed to eliminate insufficient reporting, improve inferences of efficacy/effectiveness, and better understand how outcomes may differ by setting. As described in Chapter 3, dementia care interventions themselves are often complex, involving myriad interconnected components that interact with each other and with the context and system in which they are implemented. Using the organizational framework presented in that chapter as a guide, consideration of classifying interventions at all levels (i.e., individual/family, community, policy, and societal) is warranted.

Focus on Outcomes of Greatest Importance to Persons Living with Dementia and Their Care Partners and Caregivers

In reviewing the quality of the existing evidence on dementia care interventions, one finds that most studies to date have not taken stakeholder perspectives, and the diversity of those perspectives, into account from the outset. Chapter 2 highlights the field's movement toward person-centered care; however, this term does not characterize the type of care most persons living with dementia currently receive. The broader task at hand is not only to assess the current evidence in order to decide which interventions to implement, but also to redefine the intervention development process to be more responsive to the needs of stakeholders—for example, designing interventions to address aspects of a person's well-being, including personhood, financial strain, or social isolation; imparting to caregivers the skills to better manage complex medical conditions and medications; or reevaluating payment models to provide coverage for evidence-based interventions.[1] In light of the COVID-19 pandemic, these evolving needs might also include the effects of social isolation on persons living with dementia and family care dyads, and the management of increasing medical complexity at home. In addition, a strengths-based approach (discussed in Chapter 2) is needed to examine interventions and outcome measures that focus on the strengths of persons living with dementia and their care partners and caregivers.

Outcomes that are important to persons living with dementia and their care partners and caregivers are also likely to vary depending on the age at onset and stage of disease and the needs at that time; for example, persons

[1] Presented by Laura Gitlin of Drexel University at the Care Interventions for Individuals with Dementia and Their Caregivers workshop on April 15, 2020.

in the early stage of the disease who are independent and those in later stages will have different needs. The same is true for direct care workers as well (Jennings et al., 2017) (see Chapter 5). These variations over time have implications for the design of studies with longer durations, as there may be a need to modify the outcomes examined throughout the course of the study. Moreover, it will be important to elicit and assess goals that persons living with dementia and their care partners and caregivers may have for dementia care and how these goals may change along the continuum from early- to late-stage disease (Jennings et al., 2017, 2018). Identifying these evolving person-centered goals may help determine the outcomes that matter most to stakeholders at various time points and allow researchers to better evaluate the successes and shortfalls of an intervention. For example, Jennings and colleagues (2017, 2018) report that one goal noted among persons living with dementia and caregivers in terms of accessing services and supports was being able to feel that financial resources are not a barrier to care. Another study identified days spent at home (i.e., time spent out of hospitals, postacute rehabilitation, and nursing homes) as an outcome of importance to older adults, including persons living with dementia and their caregivers (Sayer, 2016). In light of the likelihood that the needs of persons living with dementia and their care partners and caregivers will evolve over time, research is needed to develop meaningful timescales for each outcome measure with an understanding of the expected pace of change in that measure, the ability for that behavior to be sustained, and the value placed on it by participants in the intervention. Needed as well are more effective ways of involving those who will implement emerging interventions (e.g., providers, persons living with dementia, care partners, and caregivers) in the process of intervention development.

Within the set of harmonized outcomes and measures for dementia care research, a person's well-being is central. As noted in Chapters 1 and 2, this was a recurring theme highlighted among a group of persons living with dementia, care partners, and caregivers who served as advisers to the committee. Accordingly, it will be important for intervention studies to examine both the harms and benefits of an intervention, intended and unintended and for diverse stakeholders, including perspectives of future adopters. While caregiver burden was a common measure in the studies reviewed in the AHRQ systematic review, harms (e.g., elder abuse) were rarely assessed (Butler et al., 2020). Yet, Dong and colleagues (2014) report that, although 27.9–62.3 percent of older adults with dementia experience some form of psychological abuse and an estimated 3.5–23.1 percent experience physical abuse, elder abuse is often underreported in this population for a number of reasons (e.g., fear of retaliation and loss of support). Caregiver stress and burden is a common risk factor for elder abuse (Dong, 2017; Lee and Kolomer, 2005; Yan and Kwok, 2011). In a prior study of caregivers for persons living with dementia, an expert panel found that 47 percent of persons living with dementia had experienced abuse, which corresponded to caregivers' self-reported elder abuse (Wiglesworth et al., 2010). Caregiver anxiety, depressive symptoms, perceived burden, emotional status, and role limitations due to emotional problems were among the most common predictors of this abuse. "The combination of caregivers' physical assault and psychological aggression provided the best sensitivity and specificity for elder mistreatment as defined by the expert panel" (Wiglesworth et al., 2010).

Similarly, the AHRQ systematic review revealed a lack of outcomes related to harms to care partners and caregivers. For example, it is estimated that severe aggression by persons living with dementia toward care partners and caregivers takes place at a rate greater than 20 percent and may be the strongest predictor of nursing home placement (Wharton and Ford, 2014). The same experiences occur among direct care workers, including those in long-term dementia care settings, who report higher rates of emotional and physical abuse by residents compared with nurses in hospitals (Boström et al., 2012).

The added stress and burdens caused by the COVID-19 pandemic have exacerbated some of the challenges faced by both persons living with dementia and their care partners and caregivers, resulting in increased risk for new abusive situations and potential increased severity of existing abusive relationships (Makaroun et al., 2020). These include elder abuse and caregiver and self-neglect, for which tools exist to predict at-risk individuals (Dong and Simon, 2014; Wang et al., 2020). Recognizing that outcomes related to intended and unintended harms are difficult to evaluate using quantitative metrics, further investment in qualitative and mixed-method research designs may be needed to capture these outcomes.

Include Qualitative Methods in Studies That Have Quantitative Outcomes

Given the complexity of dementia and the progression of the disease and care needs over time, qualitative and mixed-method research designs are needed to better understand the experience of persons living with dementia, care partners, and caregivers with a particular intervention and the context in which the intervention was implemented. While measurement of quantitative outcomes enables pooling of results across studies, qualitative methods offer greater insight into the acceptability and feasibility of an intervention and the relevance of context to its adoption among stakeholders. For example, qualitative methods might capture the experiences and perceptions of direct care workers caring for persons living with dementia, as well as the experiences and perceptions of that care among the persons living with dementia (Houghton et al., 2016; Reilly and Houghton, 2019). Synthesized qualitative findings can be developed from a body of qualitative studies and graded using a process analogous to Grading of Recommendations Assessment, Development and Evaluation (GRADE). GRADE-CERQual (Confidence in the Evidence from Reviews of Qualitative research) is an approach that can be used to "assess how much confidence to place in findings from a qualitative evidence synthesis" using four criteria: methodological limitations, coherence, adequacy of data, and relevance (Lewin et al., 2015, 2018). Such evidence may complement the evaluation of the level of certainty of effectiveness for an intervention and help inform research, policy development, and practice.

Mixed-method research strategies have the potential to accelerate the translation of research findings into practice. As noted in Chapter 4, the hybrid effectiveness–implementation designs proposed by Curran and colleagues (2012) could help address issues related to internal and external validity and give researchers the latitude to study a range of outcomes (e.g., efficacy and implementation). Measuring these outcomes in both quantitative and qualitative ways would give researchers a better understanding of the implementation process, stakeholder perspectives, and areas for improvement (see Proctor et al., 2011). In addition, qualitative assessment of the factors outlined in the Normalization Process Theory (NPT) framework (described in Chapter 4)—coherence, cognitive participation, collective action, and reflexive monitoring—might help researchers understand how best to modify interventions as needed for different contexts and subpopulations (Murray et al., 2010).

Prior research in minority populations suggests that social and cultural context are important factors to consider (as discussed in greater detail below), but they are not commonly measured in traditional quantitative research (Brewster et al., 2019). Dementia is often perceived differently in various cultures (Dilworth-Anderson and Gibson, 2002), and substantial barriers exist in screening, diagnosing, and treating certain populations (Chin et al., 2011). Knowledge from the behavioral, social, and anthropological sciences may provide synergistic contributions to help address some of the above-noted limitations of dementia care research.

The committee acknowledges the ongoing efforts of NIH and NIA to institute new funding mechanisms that prioritize implementation science and the NIH Stage Model and align with the need for qualitative and mixed-method approaches.[2] To continue to advance work in this domain, it may be necessary to establish expert working groups to develop standards and guidance on when best to use qualitative and mixed-method designs for dementia care research.

---

[2] One such example is the NIA IMPACT (IMbedded Pragmatic Alzheimer's disease and related dementias Clinical Trials) Collaboratory. For more information, see https://impactcollaboratory.org (accessed December 11, 2020).

Use Observational Studies as a Complement to Randomized Trials

While the AHRQ systematic review analytic set included only randomized trials, high-quality observational studies can also generate useful evidence on the effectiveness of interventions (see Table 6-1). Observational studies can provide insight into the magnitude of a problem and/or risk factors that serve as a point of intervention, and offer a cost-effective way to monitor progress toward remediation of identified problems over time. The data thus obtained can serve as benchmarks for interventionists or adopters of interventions in evaluating the populations they serve.

TABLE 6-1 Overview of Randomized and Nonrandomized/Observational Study Designs at the Individual and Community Levels, with Selected Examples

	Randomized Experiments	Nonrandomized Experiments and Observational Studies
Individual Level	**Individually Randomized Trials** Randomized trials randomly assign individuals to one or more interventions, including a control, which may be standard care or some other comparator. The occurrence of an outcome is then compared between those assigned to each intervention. The key advantage of randomized trials is that the groups receiving each intervention are, on average, comparable at the time of assignment to the interventions. However, some randomized trials have strict eligibility criteria or implement interventions in highly controlled conditions and thus do not enable evaluation of the interventions' real-world effects. Pragmatic randomized trials address these issues by comparing realistic interventions in broader populations.	**Follow-Up Studies** Observational follow-up studies compare the outcomes of individuals who happen to receive the interventions of interest without the investigators' participation. Quasi-experiments (discussed further below under the community level) compare the outcomes of individuals whose interventions are assigned by the investigators but in a nonrandomized way. Because the assignment of interventions is not randomized, these designs may suffer from bias due to noncomparability between the groups receiving each intervention. Follow-up studies may be particularly useful for generalizing results for purposes of clinical practice, because they, like pragmatic randomized trials, typically include individuals that more closely represent the target population, and they occur under real-world conditions. Statistical adjustment and sensitivity analyses are generally required to handle prognostic factors that are imbalanced across intervention groups.

continued

TABLE 6-1 Continued

	Randomized Experiments	Nonrandomized Experiments and Observational Studies
Community Level	**Cluster Randomized Trials** Cluster randomized trials randomly assign groups, such as a local community or the patients seen at a specific clinic, to one or more interventions, including a control. The control may be standard care or some other comparator. Cluster randomized trials may be particularly useful for evaluating public health, health policy, or health system interventions, since decisions to implement these interventions generally are made for a group of people (e.g., a community) rather than individuals. Cluster randomized trials are also used for interventions that are likely to be learned by participants who will have frequent contact with each other.	**Quasi-Experimental Designs** Quasi-experimental designs use a nonrandom method to assign participants to groups. Common types of these designs include nonequivalent group, posttest; nonequivalent group, pre–posttest; and interrupted time series. Quasi-experimental designs are used in the evaluation of interventions, including real-world effectiveness, when random assignment is not possible, ethical, or practical. While the findings may be more generalizable than those of randomized controlled trials, these designs are limited in their ability to determine the causal relationship between the intervention and outcome measure. **Natural Experiments of Policy Interventions** "Natural experiment" is a commonly used misnomer for an observational study in which groups of individuals receive a new intervention, often because of changes in health policies. Like cluster randomized trials, natural experiments are useful to study population-level interventions (e.g., changes in payment, or examination of differences in service outcomes by models). Like all observational studies, however, natural experiments are subject to bias due to noncomparability between the intervention groups.

SOURCES: Berger et al., 2012; Craig et al., 2012; Gribbons and Herman, 1996; Lu, 2009; Moberg and Kramer, 2015; Wiegersma et al., 2001.

Numerous features of the research context for studying persons living with dementia and their care partners and caregivers—including substantial heterogeneity in outcomes that necessitates large sample sizes to achieve adequate power, the infeasibility of randomization in some settings and for some interventions, and the need for lengthy follow-up—make randomized trials difficult or infeasible to conduct. Longitudinal observational studies provide one means of generating complementary evidence for interventions that addresses these challenges (Concato et al., 2000). Such studies leverage existing or construct new cohorts to understand more precisely the risk/protective factors and potential causal mechanisms associated with the outcomes of interest. Given the rapid growth in U.S. minority populations, the construction of new representative, population-based state, regional, and national cohorts that remedy the limited diversity of existing cohorts discussed above is essential to improving the quality of the evidence base (an issue discussed in detail later in this chapter).

Finally, while the use of longitudinal observational studies has the potential to expand the evidence base, it is important that observational analyses be designed to emulate pragmatic randomized trials as closely as possible, when appropriate (Hernán and Robins, 2016). In some cases, observational studies may be used to study types of interventions (e.g., broad policy changes to reimbursement and regulations) for which pragmatic trials are not relevant (Craig et al., 2012). Further discussion of the use of these methods to assess the real-world effectiveness of an intervention is provided later in the chapter.

Commit to Comprehensive Study Reporting

The AHRQ systematic review highlights a variety of shortcomings in reporting of study results that impeded analysis. These included the need to improve and better understand fidelity in implementation, lack of reporting about the effects of the context in which an intervention was implemented, and lack of reporting on null findings or negative results and methodological approaches that did not work (Butler et al., 2020). Comprehensive study reporting would provide a richer evidence base on which to make decisions about implementation and dissemination.

Fidelity is the extent to which an intervention is administered as intended, in terms of both content and dose (Vernooij-Dassen and Moniz-Cook, 2014). An understanding of fidelity is critical to knowing the essential elements of an intervention and how it works. Problems with fidelity, regardless of the type of research, can have significant implications for the interpretation of findings, may result in a high risk of bias and the inability to replicate the study with the same level of effectiveness, and have a negative impact on translation and implementation. The inability of a study to achieve fidelity across multiple sites may be a useful indication of whether an intervention is feasible or potentially shed light on contextual effects.

One challenge reported in the AHRQ systematic review is that interventions often have been conducted in selected populations, and their effectiveness when implemented more broadly and in other groups is unclear (Butler et al., 2020). This might be the case, for example, when an intervention tailored to the needs of a first time care partner or caregiver is implemented with others who have prior experience caring for someone with dementia. Fidelity to an intervention may also vary depending on the number of care partners or caregivers a person living with dementia may have—none, one, or more than one (e.g., multiple family members taking shifts to help provide support and care to the person living with dementia).

The AHRQ systematic review found that many studies did not include detailed information on methodology outlining the delivery of the intervention, impeding an assessment of fidelity. In addition, fidelity to the intervention differed between formal and informal caregivers in the literature; measures to ensure that the intervention was delivered as designed were less likely to be used for informal caregivers.

Given the importance of implementation fidelity to understanding the effectiveness of an intervention, these are notable gaps. Furthermore, consensus is lacking in the field on the components of fidelity assessment approaches and how to measure them (Butler et al., 2020). Chapter 4 describes one conceptual framework for assessment of implementation fidelity, proposed by Carroll and colleagues (2007), which includes three areas of evaluation: (1) adherence; (2) moderators that might influence fidelity; and (3) identification of essential components of the intervention that have the most impact, which can be methodologically complex as it implies "breaking" the randomized assignment in the analysis.

The lack of standardized methods for improving implementation fidelity and for assessing how much real-world adaptation can be tolerated before fidelity is no longer realistic represents an important research need. In 2004, the Treatment Fidelity Workgroup of the National Institutes of Health Behavior Change Consortium made several recommendations for researchers to incorporate practices of treatment fidelity in their studies more consistently. The proposed strategies were related to the study design (e.g., ensure the same treatment dose across conditions); provider training (e.g., ensure provider skill acquisition); monitoring and improving the delivery of treatment (e.g., control for provider differences); receipt of treatment (e.g., ensure participant comprehension); and enactment of treatment skills (e.g., ensure participant use of cognitive skills) (Bellg et al., 2004). The adoption of similar approaches for dementia care research is needed to improve fidelity in the field.

Equally important is determining ways to better understand fidelity when its improvement may not be feasible. To this end, when interventions are implemented in real-world settings, researchers could provide a detailed report of specific adaptations made and analyze whether those differences affected the study outcomes. Also critical is examining and reporting on contextual effects, such as the care delivery system in which an intervention is delivered, and indicating whether the intervention was sustained after the study was completed. As discussed in Chapter 3, even when a community setting or system is not targeted by an intervention, the community, policy, and societal contexts in which the intervention is implemented may influence its effectiveness. Similarly, heterogeneity in study populations can contribute to variation in the observed effects of interventions. This context sensitivity contributes to the complexity of dementia care interventions and the challenges of evaluating their effectiveness, and understanding the effects of context is therefore critically important to implementation decisions. Moreover, variability in outcomes that is unattributed may lead to false conclusions about the ineffectiveness of interventions. Including and reporting on subgroup analyses/interaction testing in studies can help identify contextual effects and ultimately inform the better design of interventions and their targeting to those most likely to benefit.

To understand the contribution of contextual effects to observed variation in an intervention's effectiveness across studies, sufficient detail is needed on the intervention's implementation (how it was implemented and under which conditions). The TIDieR framework for intervention reporting (Hoffmann et al., 2014) is an extension of other reporting frameworks (e.g., CONSORT, SPIRIT) that goes beyond the description of an intervention to include contextual factors related to implementation, such as the intervention provider and setting. For large-scale research, including contextual variables in the analyses of specific interventions (e.g., Area Health Resources Files[3]) may help in better understanding outcomes. Realist review methods are increasingly being used to understand how complex public health, policy, and health services interventions work, for whom, and in which contexts (Pawson et al., 2005), and may be useful in elucidating these relationships for dementia care interventions.

One key contributor to advancing research is learning from others in the field about what has and has not worked. To this end, researchers have to commit to reporting on null findings, negative results, and methodological approaches not found to be successful. Doing so may illuminate for other researchers practices and interventions whose further implementation is not warranted (Largent and Karlawish, 2020), and, more important, is

[3] For more information on Area Health Resources Files, see https://data.hrsa.gov/topics/health-workforce/ahrf (accessed October 13, 2020).

the researcher's scientific and ethical obligation to the study participants. Yet, selective reporting of different outcomes that had a significant effect continues to bias the literature.

Critical to advancing the research enterprise, then, is addressing known barriers to reporting through the delivery of incentives and enforcement of requirements to report. While increasingly more funders are requiring researchers to report the results of their studies (NIH, 2017b), greater insights could be gained if researchers published their full protocols (e.g., in ClinicalTrials.gov) and made their data publicly available for others to review and possibly replicate. NIA, for example, is increasingly requiring data from its supported trials to be posted in repositories or consortiums for broad data sharing, when possible.[4] When data were missing or not found to be significant, researchers could provide additional insights as to why that was the case (e.g., readiness of the researchers, lack of community buy-in or trust). Methodology papers detailing the delivery characteristics, fidelity, and setting (e.g., nursing homes, residential care facilities, adult day centers, individual homes) of an intervention might help address some of those questions.

According to the AHRQ systematic review,

> dementia care research has been slow to incorporate key elements of rigorous intervention design. Until relatively recently, many dementia care intervention studies were not held to preregistration of trials, data safety and monitoring boards, or other standards more common in other areas of clinical science including reporting standards (e.g. the Consolidated Standards of Reporting Trials [CONSORT] statement). (Butler et al., 2020, p. 109)

Although NIH requires preregistration of all the clinical trials it funds (NIH, 2017a), this practice is variable across studies, and it is unclear how closely registration for trials is followed. In addition, the registration of observational studies remains an evolving area. Much of the early work in the field occurred before trial registration was mandated or the revised 2010 CONSORT standards existed, all of which contributes to the challenges in this field's evidence base.

PRIORITIZING INCLUSIVE RESEARCH

A critical aspect of strengthening the evidence base for care interventions for persons living with dementia, care partners, and caregivers is ensuring that the research is representative and generalizable across popu-

[4] For more information on NIA Guidance for Sharing Data and Other Resources, see https://www.hhs.gov/guidance/document/nia-specific-funding-policies (accessed December 9, 2020).

lations. To this end, studies must have broadly inclusive research teams equipped with knowledge and experience working with underrepresented populations and in different settings; develop and adhere to recruitment strategies targeted at increasing the representation of racially, ethnically, culturally, linguistically, sexually, and socioeconomically diverse participants; and use study designs that support inclusivity. Strengthening the evidence base to advance the ultimate goal of improving well-being for all will require greater investments in increasing diversity across the entire research enterprise (e.g., researchers, study participants, and stakeholders), along with accountability measures to assess progress.

Conduct Studies Using Broadly Inclusive Research Teams

A lived experience cannot be taught. Diverse, multidisciplinary research teams are needed to ensure that team members collectively have insights into and sensitivity to different perspectives and cultures. Moreover, resources are needed to address knowledge and readiness gaps between researchers and stakeholders in the community. Researchers often do not know how to apply effective interventions in different populations and have not addressed fundamental questions before attempting to do so (Skinner et al., 2018). For example, how did the researchers conceptualize the problem in a social context, do they understand the social determinants of health, do they have knowledge of intersectionality and the optimal recruitment strategies for each targeted population, do they measure the intended and unintended consequences and harms of the intervention (Dong et al., 2014), and do they have the appropriate tools and training to apply the study methodology in diverse populations?

Before launching a study, then, researchers need to understand the people living in the community, as well as their history, culture, and resources. This point applies also to language and the use of terminology that resonates with the targeted population (e.g., "care partner" versus "caregiver") (see Chapter 1), as well as an understanding of how different subpopulations may prioritize different needs. For example, in the Kame Project—a study designed to examine the rates of and risk factors for dementia and its subtypes among a Japanese American population in Seattle, Washington—the researchers took several steps to tailor the study to meet the needs of the community. These steps included hiring staff from the community, engaging a community advisory board, and adapting all of the study tools and instruments to ensure linguistic and cultural understanding (Graves et al., 1996). Understanding readiness within the community of interest is essential as well, as is determining what participants hope to gain from the study and how the researchers can engage them to be part of the research team to gain a better understanding of their cultural values, belief systems, and what is important to them (e.g., serving on advisory boards). Once these questions have been answered, the researchers can determine what theory will drive the study, and then the specific methodology (Dilworth-Anderson et al., 2020).

Include Racially, Ethnically, Culturally, Linguistically, Sexually, and Socioeconomically Diverse Participants, and Assess Disparities in Access and Outcomes

As the racial and ethnic diversity of the U.S. population continues to rise (Frey, 2020; U.S. Census Bureau, 2020), it is projected that nearly half of Americans aged 65 or older will not be non-Hispanic whites by 2060 (U.S. Census Bureau, 2012). This demographic shift has clear implications for research on aging. For example, it is well known that racial and ethnic minorities (e.g., African Americans/Blacks, Latinos/Hispanics, American Indians/Alaska Natives) have a higher prevalence and incidence of Alzheimer's disease and other dementias compared with older non-Hispanic whites, as well as different caregiver patterns and use of formal care (Dilworth-Anderson et al., 2008; Mayeda et al., 2016; Pinquart and Sörensen, 2011; Steenland et al., 2016). Yet, these populations are disproportionately excluded from dementia care research, as are low-income persons living with dementia and their care partners and caregivers (Dilworth-Anderson et al., 2020; Quiñones et al., 2020).

The AHRQ systematic review highlights this limitation, observing that few studies examined racial or ethnic differences (including subpopulations) and that culturally sensitive or culturally adapted interventions were rare (Butler et al., 2020). As noted in Chapter 5, the REACH II intervention and its adaptations were among the few interventions conducted in racially and ethnically diverse populations, delivered in multiple languages, and implemented in low-income communities or with low-income participants (Belle et al., 2006; Burgio et al., 2009; Cheung et al., 2014; Cho et al., 2019; Czaja et al., 2013, 2018; Lykens et al., 2014). Furthermore, the AHRQ review identified few interventions designed for low-resource areas or rural or tribal communities, other than pilot and small-sample studies, and no studies looked at LGBTQ populations or persons with Down syndrome with dementia (Butler et al., 2020). In short, there remains a critical gap in the development and implementation of dementia care interventions tailored to and driven by the needs of persons living with dementia, care partners, and caregivers from underrepresented groups and low-resource areas, as well as persons living with dementia who do not have care partners or caregivers.

To advance the field, it will be important to understand the cultural aspect of dementia and caregiving in diverse populations and the resultant implications for methodological approaches and implementation (Apesoa-Varano et al., 2015; Chin et al., 2011). During the committee's public workshop, J. Neil Henderson from the University of Minnesota noted that a better understanding of culture is needed in terms of designing and implementing care interventions.[5] For example, some ethnocultural and indigenous populations whose numbers are small may be excluded from studies because of demands for large sample sizes. RCTs may also be unwelcomed in such communities because of the nature of the research design with respect to dividing the population into intervention and control groups. In such cases, delayed-start study designs used in other therapeutic areas, in which all study participants receive the intervention but at different time points, may be more appropriate (Crews et al., 2019; D'Agostino, 2009; Liu-Seifert et al., 2015; Tobe et al., 2014). Henderson noted that the term "culture" is often used incorrectly as a proxy when referring to minority populations, and he emphasized the importance of thinking about culture broadly as a process of adapting to life situations using precepts, beliefs, and values.[6] He added that all people conduct caregiving in both macrocultural (e.g., the United States being a highly individualistic and independent society) and microcultural (e.g., cross-generational caregiving) systems. He stressed the critical importance of having people on research teams with deep knowledge of those cultural systems (including intragroup variance) who are involved in the study from the outset.

To achieve true progress in dementia care research, NIH will need to assume greater administrative accountability for ensuring increased representation of racial and ethnic minorities in research studies. The NIH Revitalization Act of 1993[7] amends the Public Health Service Act to incorporate a mandate for the inclusion of minorities in all NIH clinical research; however, progress on carrying out this mandate remains slow (Oh et al., 2015). The law was created in part as a result of the U.S. Public Health Service Syphilis Study at Tuskegee, in which African Americans were recruited for a study aimed at ensuring harm (Rencher and Wolf, 2013). Lack of adherence to this law has led to low percentages of underrepresented minorities in dementia clinical trials, representing a missed scientific opportunity to fully understand the effectiveness and safety of interventions in these populations, a gap that may exacerbate existing health disparities (Gilmore-Bykovskyi et al., 2018; Oh et al., 2015; Quiñones et al., 2020). Accordingly, follow-through by NIH and other

[5] Presented by J. Neil Henderson of the University of Minnesota at the Care Interventions for Individuals with Dementia and Their Caregivers workshop on April 15, 2020.

[6] Presented by J. Neil Henderson of the University of Minnesota at the Care Interventions for Individuals with Dementia and Their Caregivers workshop on April 15, 2020.

[7] National Institutes of Health Revitalization Act of 1993, Public Law 103-43, 103 Cong. (June 10, 1993).

funding sources on grant awardees' recruitment and retention strategies is crucial (Dilworth-Anderson and Cohen, 2010; Dilworth-Anderson et al., 2005; Gilmore-Bykovskyi et al., 2019).

To close this gap, further training (i.e., retooling) is needed on learning and applying inclusive approaches in recruitment and on the impact of structural/system-level factors on recruitment approaches and successes (Dilworth-Anderson and Cohen, 2010; Hamel et al., 2016; Williams and Corbie Smith, 2006). Such retooling can enable researchers to learn how to adapt, revise, and create new approaches to the recruitment and retention of diverse populations. It prepares researchers to use inclusive approaches to recruitment and retention of diverse populations in their research at both the conceptual and methodological levels, including thinking about and defining a problem and recruiting participants to help understand the problem. Such an approach goes beyond diversity to emphasize shared interest in and representation (inclusion) by researchers and participants in the research process. There are ongoing efforts to address this challenge at NIH and NIA, including the National Strategy for Recruitment and Participation in Alzheimer's and Related Dementia Clinical Research,[8] launched in 2018 (NIA, n.d.), and recruitment strategies of the Health and Retirement Study (Ofstedal and Weir, 2011). Nonetheless, progress remains slow.

Recognizing that a greater proportion of older adults reside in rural and remote settings than in urban environments (Smith and Trevelyan, 2019), greater attention to rural and low-resource areas is also needed (Prince et al., 2015). As noted above, few interventions considered in the AHRQ systematic review were designed for such areas, which therefore represent a critical gap in the implementation of care interventions to meet the needs of persons living with dementia, care partners, and caregivers. Closing this gap is a priority for NIA, as demonstrated by its funding opportunities and recent initiative to establish an Interdisciplinary Network on Rural Population Health and Aging,[9] and continued efforts in this area are critical. In addition, U.S. Department of Veterans Affairs (VA) populations and safety net clinics may be another key target group setting for dementia care research.

Use Study Designs That Support Inclusivity

To address the diversity gaps detailed above, researchers need to use study designs that allow for inclusivity and increase the generalizability of research findings. Given the limitations of RCTs, the incorporation of other

---

[8] For more information, see https://www.nia.nih.gov/research/recruitment-strategy (accessed October 20, 2020).

[9] For more information, see https://sites.psu.edu/inrpha (accessed November 10, 2020).

study designs, such as those discussed earlier in this chapter (e.g., quasi-experimental or longitudinal, well-designed observational studies; adaptive trial designs), is necessary to better understand whether an intervention will be effective in different subpopulations and settings. Intervention studies need to be designed with the goal of dissemination in mind, with consideration given to the potential for application in real-world care delivery and residential settings and in different cultural contexts (Damschroder et al., 2009; Green et al., 2009). As noted previously, including people from those different contexts and within the community in the study design can ensure the acceptability and feasibility of an intervention. The AHRQ systematic review notes that non-U.S.-based research may offer insights on future intervention adaptations for persons living with dementia, care partners, and caregivers with immigrant or related racial/ethnic heritages (Butler et al., 2020).

The Lancet Commission has reported that many risk factors for dementia cluster around inequalities that disproportionately affect minority and vulnerable populations, and emphasizes the need to tackle these inequalities through "not only health promotion but also societal action to improve the circumstances in which people live their lives" (Livingston et al., 2020a). For example, it has been shown that institutional racism is a factor in the social determinants of health that put minority populations at greater risk for disease, and also makes it more difficult to support and implement interventions in health systems (Brondolo et al., 2009; Chin et al., 2011; Phelan and Link, 2015). To address and help mitigate such inequalities through the continuum from prevention to late-stage care, a focus on inclusive research for dementia care interventions is needed as a complement to focusing on preventable risk factors.

ASSESSING REAL-WORLD EFFECTIVENESS

In assessing the evidence base for dementia care interventions in the context of determining readiness for broad dissemination and implementation, the AHRQ systematic review was guided by the NIH Stage Model for Behavioral Interventions (Butler et al., 2020). This model delineates the full continuum of intervention research, ranging from basic science research and new intervention design to dissemination and implementation research (Onken et al., 2014). Interventions further along in that continuum (at Stage III or higher) have been studied under more real-world conditions and are more likely to be ready for broad dissemination. For the majority of interventions reviewed, however, the AHRQ review found few instances of progression along the NIH Stage Model beyond the basic explanatory stage (Stage III) (Butler et al., 2020), indicating little evidence of real-world effectiveness. As noted earlier in this chapter, these pilot studies and studies with small sample sizes in the AHRQ systematic review are valuable for assessing feasibility or proof of concept. To be ready for broad dissemination and implementation, however, research must advance interventions further along the Stage Model and generate evidence about their application to individuals, communities, and systems. This section examines approaches to addressing this need.

Improve the Assessment of Individual-Level Interventions by Leveraging Complementary Study Methodologies

The framework for dementia care interventions presented in Chapter 3 depicts the various levels at which interventions may be implemented—at the individual, community, and policy levels. As discussed earlier in this chapter, much of the focus on interventions in the field has been on those targeting individual persons living with dementia, care partners, and caregivers. The effectiveness of these individual-level interventions can be assessed using randomized trials and observational studies that emulate randomized trials.

Randomized trials, and especially pragmatic trials, are helpful to establish effectiveness in the real world (see above). In some cases, pragmatic trials may be efficiently embedded in health care and other support delivery systems to leverage electronic health records (EHRs) for recruitment (to shorten enrollment times and improve recruitment of specific racial/ethnic groups or vulnerable populations), for data collection, or even as part of an intervention (e.g., alerts). However, the limitations of these trials need to be recognized. Although pragmatic trials are tested in real-world settings, they are still subject to contextual challenges that can impact the implementation and sustainability of the intervention (e.g., high caregiver turnover). Because randomized trials are logistically complex and expensive, they often have relatively small sample sizes and follow-up durations. As a result, they may yield imprecise effect estimates over short time horizons (Sim, 2019) or use proxy measures in lieu of clinically relevant outcomes (Krauss, 2018). In addition, failure to adhere to the trial protocol may obscure the effectiveness of otherwise promising interventions (if only adherence could be increased). That is, the usual intention-to-treat effect estimates need to be complemented with per-protocol effect estimates that adjust for deviations from the trial protocol (Hernán and Robins, 2017).

Observational studies may overcome some of the limitations of randomized trials, but they are vulnerable to several biases. First, the lack of randomized assignment may lead to noncomparable groups (Lu, 2009). The design of observational studies needs to incorporate the measurement of prognostic factors that may be imbalanced between intervention groups and that will have to be adjusted for in the statistical analyses. Second, a naïve analysis of observational data may lead to serious biases, such as selection bias and immortal time bias. By designing observational analyses with the explicit goal of emulating a (hypothetical) pragmatic trial—the target trial—these biases can be reduced (Hernán et al., 2016). At the very least, sound observational analyses may help design better randomized trials.

Expand the Focus on Community/Policy-Level Interventions Using a Broad Set of Research Methodologies

Because much of the focus of dementia care research has been on interventions applied to individuals, the AHRQ systematic review includes a paucity of evidence for interventions applied to communities or to the entire system. Estimating the effectiveness of the latter interventions is difficult, especially when they are implemented in parallel with individual-level interventions, as it can be difficult to link many distal processes of care to desired outcomes (NQF, 2014). Improving the evidence for these kinds of interventions will necessitate methodologies other than those used to study individual interventions.

Cluster randomized trials (discussed earlier in this chapter) can be used to quantify the effectiveness of interventions implemented in communities ("clusters"). Observational studies that do not require individual-level data can also be used to evaluate these types of interventions or to help design cluster randomized trials. For example, ecological studies can be used to generate hypotheses that can later be studied in cluster randomized trials, and so-called quasi-experimental studies can estimate effects of a specific intervention by comparing the changes in outcomes over time between the intervention and control groups (e.g., using difference-in-difference analyses when the assumptions of the method hold).

Extreme instances of community-level interventions are those that are applied to an entire system in the form of new policies (e.g., payment change; state regulations; training grocery store clerks and bank tellers in the community to understand, recognize, and assist customers living with dementia to improve quality of life for them and their care partners and caregivers). The effect of system-wide interventions generally cannot be studied via randomized trials or observational studies that emulate randomized trials, and often cannot be studied using ecological or quasi-experimental approaches. Estimating the effects of system-wide interventions may therefore require the construction of policy models, and to this end, researchers can apply the modeling expertise developed in other health fields to expand their focus to system-wide interventions.

Address Key Factors Needed to Assess Real-World Effectiveness

As discussed in Chapter 4, decisions to implement interventions depend not only on evidence of efficacy from controlled research studies but also on factors that influence the feasibility of implementation (e.g., workforce needs, cost, alignment with current workflow), which will influence the intervention's effectiveness in real-world settings. These considerations can be incorporated into decisions on whether interventions are ready to move into pragmatic trials (Baier et al., 2019) or should be recommended for dissemination and implementation (Moberg et al., 2018). As discussed in detail in Chapter 5, in considering whether either of the intervention types with low-strength evidence of effectiveness identified in the AHRQ systematic review were ready for broad dissemination and implementation, the committee evaluated the evidence using the GRADE (Grading of Recommendations Assessment, Development and Evaluation) Evidence to Decision framework and noted significant gaps related to the quality and heterogeneity of the evidence. Such gaps will need to be addressed in future research to better inform the identification of interventions ready for broad dissemination and to meet the information needs of stakeholders (e.g., systems providing services and supports, payers, policy makers) responsible for making decisions about implementation and coverage of dementia care interventions.

NIA has already started to move in this direction, as exemplified by the development of the NIH Stage Model, as noted earlier in this chapter. In some cases, focused investigation of particular factors that are critical for assessing real-world effectiveness (e.g., financial constraints) could be conducted through studies that fit within NIH's current R01 framework, incremental steps that would extend the R21 (exploratory/developmental grants) and R34 (grant planning program) approaches, or funding of replication studies.[10] NIA could expand this approach, for example, by providing a road map for researchers offering funding support for each stage of the NIH Stage Model tailored to the unique challenges inherent in dementia care research and the many opportunities for future research identified in this chapter.

Approaches to addressing such gaps may include embedded pragmatic trials (which often involve stakeholders responsible for the adoption of interventions) and observational analyses carried out in practice settings that implement the interventions of interest (or by a third-party organization). In particular, a network of community-benefit organizations could help provide practical pragmatic, real-world information about the effectiveness, consistency, and impact of different organizations and service

[10] For more information, see https://grants.nih.gov/grants/funding/funding_program.htm (accessed December 11, 2020).

providers, similar to a practiced-based research network.[11] Observational studies can also be used to examine the relevance of policy and payment changes by geographies and organizational characteristics. The NIA IMPACT Collaboratory is building capacity to conduct embedded pragmatic clinical trials (ePCTs) to accelerate the translation of evidence-based interventions into practice as well (Mitchell et al., 2020).

As discussed previously, engaging the full range of stakeholders who will be using and implementing an intervention (e.g., persons living with dementia, care partners, and caregivers; community-based organizations; long-term services and supports providers; managed care organizations; health systems) in the design and evaluation of interventions can help ensure that implementation considerations (e.g., feasibility) are taken into account from the beginning and that interventions are appropriately tailored for the populations and contexts in which they will be implemented. This continues to be a priority for NIA, as demonstrated through the triennial National Research Summit on Care, Services, and Supports for Persons with Dementia and Their Caregivers, which engages a broad range of stakeholders, and the requests for applications emanating directly from those meetings.[12]

As discussed earlier, it is important to have evidence-based interventions that meet the needs of persons living with dementia, care partners, and caregivers at various time points in terms of the stage of disease and length of caregiving time.[13] Community-based participatory research and community-partnered participatory research are existing models that support this kind of partnering. These models, which emphasize that the community of study and academic researchers are equal partners in the design, implementation, and dissemination of interventions (IOM, 2000; Viswanathan et al., 2004; Wells and Jones, 2009), have been applied in research with persons living with dementia, care partners, and caregivers, including a rural and remote dementia care program (e.g., Morgan et al., 2014). Morgan and colleagues note that stakeholder partnerships enhanced the quality, relevance, application, and sustainability of the research, which led to the adoption of a telehealth-delivered frontotemporal dementia support group model for a province-wide program in Canada and the transfer of the Rural and Remote Memory Clinic research project to a sustained program funded by the province's ministry of health (Morgan et al., 2014).

Finally, while cost-effectiveness was beyond of the scope of the AHRQ systematic review and this committee did not conduct such an analysis, sev-

[11] Presented by Patrick Courneya of HealthPartners at the Care Interventions for Individuals with Dementia and Their Caregivers workshop on April 15, 2020.

[12] For more information, see https://aspe.hhs.gov/national-research-summit-care-services-and-supports-persons-dementia-and-their-caregivers (accessed December 11, 2020).

[13] Presented by Kathleen Kelly of Family Caregiver Alliance at the Care Interventions for Individuals with Dementia and Their Caregivers workshop on April 15, 2020.

eral dementia care interventions have demonstrated benefits with respect to various types of utilization and overall Medicare costs, including research supported through Center for Medicare & Medicaid Innovation (CMMI) Health Care Innovation Awards (NORC at the University of Chicago, 2016). For example, the University of California, Los Angeles, Alzheimer's and Dementia Care program observed significant reductions in hospitalizations for ambulatory care–sensitive conditions and 30-day readmissions, a 25 percent lower rate of nursing home placement, and a lower average cost of care among study participants (NORC at the University of Chicago, 2016).

RECOMMENDATIONS

While much progress has been made toward expanding and improving dementia care research, progress to date has been insufficient to meet the needs of the nation's aging society with its increased numbers of persons needing services that advance their well-being. The evidence for care interventions for persons living with dementia, care partners, and caregivers remains complex and is lacking as the result of a number of methodological and implementation challenges. Over time, criteria for assessing the rigor and validity of research are becoming more standardized and rigorous, but this progress is not yet fully reflected in the overall body of literature assessed in the AHRQ systematic review. This progress should be encouraged, along with additional methodological improvements needed across the research enterprise to strengthen the rigor and representativeness of the evidence base for dementia care interventions at multiple levels, as well as the evidence base on the effect of interventions under real-world conditions.

The committee also emphasizes the significant impact the COVID-19 pandemic has had on quality of life for persons living with dementia and their care partners and caregivers, as well as the implications for research (e.g., challenges to study recruitment), implementation (e.g., decreased face-to-face interactions), and dissemination. This issue will require attention in the months and years to come.

The methodological improvements outlined in this chapter cannot all be achieved in a single study, but rather apply collectively across research in the field. In this context, it is essential for researchers, NIA, and other interested organizations to consider the specific actions they each can take to contribute to advancing dementia care research. Ensuring that well-being and personhood, as well as inclusive research, remain central is the responsibility of all.

RECOMMENDATION 3: *Use strong, pragmatic, and informative methodologies.*
When requesting applications and identifying funding priorities for research on care interventions for persons living with dementia and their care partners and caregivers, the National Institute on Aging and other interested organizations should prioritize strong, pragmatic, and informative methodologies that take account of this complex domain, including studies that

- ensure a balanced portfolio of short- and longer-term studies with sufficient sample size;
- use a harmonized core of outcomes and a taxonomy of interventions to enable pooling of study findings;
- focus on outcomes of greatest priority to persons living with dementia and their care partners and caregivers, including intended and unintended benefits and harms, across the continuum of early- through late-stage dementia;
- include qualitative methods in studies that have quantitative outcomes;
- use observational study methods to complement randomized trials; and
- commit to comprehensive study reporting to enable improving and better understanding fidelity, studying context effects, and learning from negative results and unsuccessful methodological approaches.

RECOMMENDATION 4: *Prioritize inclusive research.*
When funding research on care interventions for persons living with dementia and their care partners and caregivers, the National Institutes of Health (NIH) and other interested organizations should prioritize research that promotes equity, diversity, and inclusion across the full range of populations and communities affected by dementia through studies that

- are conducted by broadly inclusive research teams;
- include racially, ethnically, culturally, linguistically, sexually, and socioeconomically diverse participants by requiring adherence to the NIH Revitalization Act of 1993, and assess disparities in access and outcomes; and
- use study designs that support inclusivity.

RECOMMENDATION 5: *Assess real-world effectiveness.*
When funding research on care interventions for persons living with dementia, care partners, and caregivers, the National Institutes of Health, the Agency for Healthcare Research and Quality, the Centers for Medicare & Medicaid Services, the Administration for Community Living, and other interested organizations should support research capable of providing the evidence that will ultimately be needed to make inclusive decisions and implement interventions in the real world, including studies that, to the extent possible,

- **improve the assessment of individual-level interventions by leveraging complementary study methodologies;**
- **expand the focus on community/policy-level interventions using a broad set of research methodologies; and**
- **address key factors (e.g., space, human resources, work redesign, and adaptations) that need to be taken into account to assess the real-world effectiveness of these interventions.**

FINAL THOUGHTS

To address the long-standing and urgent imperative to better support persons living with dementia and their care partners and caregivers in living as well as possible, there continues to be a critical need to build a more robust and useful evidence base. Studying dementia care interventions is challenging and complex, and the body of evidence is complicated to interpret. Two types of interventions are supported by sufficient evidence to warrant implementation in real-world settings, along with evaluation to continue to expand the evidence base. These interventions are practical instantiations of many of the core components of care, supports, and services, discussed in Chapter 2, that are needed to promote the well-being of persons living with dementia and their care partners and caregivers. Given current major deficits in the care, services, and supports that are available now, providing these interventions to those who could benefit would be a step forward. Yet, this is not a final answer. It is important that research continue to develop and evaluate other potentially promising interventions, many of which have shown some signal of benefit. The committee's recommendations provide a path forward for building a more robust and useful evidence base by employing cutting-edge methods that are rigorous, most informative for this domain, inclusive, and equitable, and can yield critical information for real-world implementation. These exciting approaches can be implemented throughout the dementia care field, including by early-career researchers and others who want to harness new approaches to make a difference in addressing this critical societal need and better supporting persons living with dementia and their care partners and caregivers in living as well as possible.

REFERENCES

Apesoa-Varano, E. C., Y. Tang-Feldman, S. C. Reinhard, R. Choula, and H. M. Young. 2015. Multi-cultural caregiving and caregiver interventions: A look back and a call for future action. *Generations* 39(4):39–48.

Baier, R. R., E. Jutkowitz, S. L. Mitchell, E. McCreedy, and V. Mor. 2019. Readiness assessment for pragmatic trials (RAPT): A model to assess the readiness of an intervention for testing in a pragmatic trial. *BMC Medical Research Methodology* 19(1):156.

Belle, S. H., L. Burgio, R. Burns, D. Coon, S. J. Czaja, D. Gallagher-Thompson, L. N. Gitlin, J. Klinger, K. M. Koepke, C. C. Lee, J. Martindale-Adams, L. Nichols, R. Schulz, S. Stahl, A. Stevens, L. Winter, and S. Zhang. 2006. Enhancing the quality of life of dementia caregivers from different ethnic or racial groups: A randomized, controlled trial. *Annals of Internal Medicine* 145(10):727–738.

Bellg, A. J., B. Borrelli, B. Resnick, J. Hecht, D. S. Minicucci, M. Ory, G. Ogedegbe, D. Orwig, D. Ernst, and S. Czajkowski. 2004. Enhancing treatment fidelity in health behavior change studies: Best practices and recommendations from the NIH behavior change consortium. *Health Psychology* 23(5):443–451.

Berger, M. L., N. Dreyer, F. Anderson, A. Towse, A. Sedrakyan, and S. L. Normand. 2012. Prospective observational studies to assess comparative effectiveness: The ISPOR good research practices task force report. *Value in Health* 15(2):217–230.

Boström, A. M., J. E. Squires, A. Mitchell, A. E. Sales, and C. A. Estabrooks. 2012. Workplace aggression experienced by frontline staff in dementia care. *Journal of Clinical Nursing* 21(9–10):1453–1465.

Brewster, P., L. Barnes, M. Haan, J. K. Johnson, J. J. Manly, A. M. Nápoles, R. A. Whitmer, L. Carvajal-Carmona, D. Early, S. Farias, E. R. Mayeda, R. Melrose, O. L. Meyer, A. Zeki Al Hazzouri, L. Hinton, and D. Mungas. 2019. Progress and future challenges in aging and diversity research in the United States. *Alzheimer's & Dementia* 15(7):995–1003.

Brondolo, E., L. C. Gallo, and H. F. Myers. 2009. Race, racism and health: Disparities, mechanisms, and interventions. *Journal of Behavioral Medicine* 32(1):1.

Burgio, L. D., I. B. Collins, B. Schmid, T. Wharton, D. McCallum, and J. Decoster. 2009. Translating the REACH caregiver intervention for use by area agency on aging personnel: The REACH OUT program. *Gerontologist* 49(1):103–116.

Butler, M., J. E. Gaugler, K. M. C. Talley, H. I. Abdi, P. J. Desai, S. Duval, M. L. Forte, V. A. Nelson, W. Ng, J. M. Ouellette, E. Ratner, J. Saha, T. Shippee, B. L. Wagner, T. J. Wilt, and L. Yeshi. 2020. Care interventions for people living with dementia and their caregivers. *Comparative Effectiveness Review No. 231*. Rockville, MD: Agency for Healthcare Research and Quality. doi: 10.23970/AHRQEPCCER231.

Carroll, C., M. Patterson, S. Wood, A. Booth, J. Rick, and S. Balain. 2007. A conceptual framework for implementation fidelity. *Implementation Science* 2(1):40.

Cheung, K. S., B. H. Lau, P. W. Wong, A. Y. Leung, V. W. Lou, G. M. Chan, and R. Schulz. 2014. Multicomponent intervention on enhancing dementia caregiver well-being and reducing behavioral problems among Hong Kong Chinese: A translational study based on REACH II. *International Journal of Geriatric Psychiatry* 30(5):460–469.

Chin, A. L., S. Negash, and R. Hamilton. 2011. Diversity and disparity in dementia: The impact of ethnoracial differences in Alzheimer disease. *Alzheimer Disease and Associated Disorders* 25(3):187–195.

Cho, J., S. Luk-Jones, D. R. Smith, and A. B. Stevens. 2019. Evaluation of REACH-TX: A community-based approach to the REACH II intervention. *Innovation in Aging* 3(3):igz022.

Concato, J., N. Shah, and R. I. Horwitz. 2000. Randomized, controlled trials, observational studies, and the hierarchy of research designs. *New England Journal of Medicine* 342(25):1887–1892.

Craig, P., C. Cooper, D. Gunnell, S. Haw, K. Lawson, S. Macintyre, D. Ogilvie, M. Petticrew, B. Reeves, M. Sutton, and S. Thompson. 2012. Using natural experiments to evaluate population health interventions: New medical research council guidance. *Journal of Epidemiology and Community Health* 66(12):1182.

Crews, D. C., A. M. Delaney, J. L. Walker Taylor, T. K. M. Cudjoe, M. Nkimbeng, L. Roberts, J. Savage, A. Evelyn-Gustave, J. Roth, D. Han, L. L. Boyér, R. J. Thorpe, D. L. Roth, L. N. Gitlin, and S. L. Szanton. 2019. Pilot intervention addressing social support and functioning of low socioeconomic status older adults with ESRD: The seniors optimizing community integration to advance better living with ESRD (SOCIABLE) study. *Kidney Medicine* 1(1):13–20.

Curran, G. M., M. Bauer, B. Mittman, J. M. Pyne, and C. Stetler. 2012. Effectiveness-implementation hybrid designs: Combining elements of clinical effectiveness and implementation research to enhance public health impact. *Medical Care* 50(3):217–226.

Czaja, S. J., D. Loewenstein, R. Schulz, S. N. Nair, and D. Perdomo. 2013. A videophone psychosocial intervention for dementia caregivers. *The American Journal of Geriatric Psychiatry* 21(11):1071–1081.

Czaja, S. J., C. C. Lee, D. Perdomo, D. Loewenstein, M. Bravo, J. H. Moxley, and R. Schulz. 2018. Community REACH: An implementation of an evidence-based caregiver program. *Gerontologist* 58(2):e130–e137.

D'Agostino, R. B., Sr. 2009. The delayed-start study design. *New England Journal of Medicine* 361(13):1304–1306.

Damschroder, L. J., D. C. Aron, R. E. Keith, S. R. Kirsh, J. A. Alexander, and J. C. Lowery. 2009. Fostering implementation of health services research findings into practice: A consolidated framework for advancing implementation science. *Implementation Science* 4(1):50.

Dilworth-Anderson, P., and M. D. Cohen. 2010. Beyond diversity to inclusion: Recruitment and retention of diverse groups in Alzheimer research. *Alzheimer Disease and Associated Disorders* 24(Suppl):S14–S18.

Dilworth-Anderson, P., and B. E. Gibson. 2002. The cultural influence of values, norms, meanings, and perceptions in understanding dementia in ethnic minorities. *Alzheimer's Disease and Associated Disorders* 16:S56–S63.

Dilworth-Anderson, P., S. Thaker, and J. M. D. Burke. 2005. Recruitment strategies for studying dementia in later life among diverse cultural groups. *Alzheimer Disease and Associated Disorders* 19(4).

Dilworth-Anderson, P., H. C. Hendrie, J. J. Manly, A. S. Khachaturian, and S. Fazio. 2008. Diagnosis and assessment of Alzheimer's disease in diverse populations. *Alzheimer's & Dementia* 4(4):305–309.

Dilworth-Anderson, P., H. Moon, and M. P. Aranda. 2020. Dementia caregiving research: Expanding and reframing the lens of diversity, inclusivity, and intersectionality. *Gerontologist* 60(5):797–805.

Dong, X. 2017. *Elder abuse: Research, practice and policy*, 1st ed. Springer International Publishing.

Dong, X., and M. A. Simon. 2014. Vulnerability risk index profile for elder abuse in a community-dwelling. *Journal of the American Geriatrics Society* 62(1):10–15.

Dong, X., R. Chen, and M. A. Simon. 2014. Elder abuse and dementia: A review of the research and health policy. *Health Affairs* 33(4):642–649.

Emsley, R., G. Dunn, and I. R. White. 2009. Mediation and moderation of treatment effects in randomised controlled trials of complex interventions. *Statistical Methods in Medical Research* 19(3):237–270.

Frey, W. H. 2020. *The nation is diversifying even faster than predicted, according to new census data.* https://www.brookings.edu/research/new-census-data-shows-the-nation-is-diversifying-even-faster-than-predicted (accessed August 12, 2020).

Gaugler, J. E., E. Jutkowitz, T. P. Shippee, and M. Brasure. 2017. Consistency of dementia caregiver intervention classification: An evidence-based synthesis. *International Psychogeriatrics* 29(1):19–30.

Gilmore-Bykovskyi, A., R. Johnson, L. Walljasper, L. Block, and N. Werner. 2018. Underreporting of gender and race/ethnicity differences in NIH-funded dementia caregiver support interventions. *American Journal of Alzheimer's Disease and Other Dementias* 33(3):145–152.

Gilmore-Bykovskyi, A. L., Y. Jin, C. Gleason, S. Flowers-Benton, L. M. Block, P. Dilworth-Anderson, L. L. Barnes, M. N. Shah, and M. Zuelsdorff. 2019. Recruitment and retention of underrepresented populations in Alzheimer's disease research: A systematic review. *Alzheimer's & Dementia: Translational Research & Clinical Interventions* 5:751–770.

Gitlin, L. N., N. Hodgson, E. Jutkowitz, and L. Pizzi. 2010. The cost-effectiveness of a nonpharmacologic intervention for individuals with dementia and family caregivers: The tailored activity program. *American Journal of Geriatric Psychiatry* 18(6):510–519.

Graves, A. B., E. B. Larson, S. D. Edland, J. D. Bowen, W. C. McCormick, S. M. McCurry, M. M. Rice, A. Wenzlow, and J. M. Uomoto. 1996. Prevalence of dementia and its subtypes in the Japanese American population of King County, Washington State: The Kame Project. *American Journal of Epidemiology* 144(8):760–771.

Green, L. W., J. M. Ottoson, C. García, and R. A. Hiatt. 2009. Diffusion theory and knowledge dissemination, utilization, and integration in public health. *Annual Review of Public Health* 30:151–174.

Gribbons, B., and J. Herman. 1996. True and quasi-experimental designs. *Practical Assessment, Research, and Evaluation* 5(1):14.

Hamel, L. M., L. A. Penner, T. L. Albrecht, E. Heath, C. K. Gwede, and S. Eggly. 2016. Barriers to clinical trial enrollment in racial and ethnic minority patients with cancer. *Cancer Control* 23(4):327–337.

Hernán, M. A., and J. M. Robins. 2016. Using big data to emulate a target trial when a randomized trial is not available. *American Journal of Epidemiology* 183(8):758–764.

Hernán, M. A., and J. M. Robins. 2017. Per-protocol analyses of pragmatic trials. *New England Journal of Medicine* 377(14):1391–1398.

Hernán, M. A., B. C. Sauer, S. Hernández-Díaz, R. Platt, and I. Shrier. 2016. Specifying a target trial prevents immortal time bias and other self-inflicted injuries in observational analyses. *Journal of Clinical Epidemiology* 79:70–75.

HHS (U.S. Department of Health and Human Services). 2018. *Report to the National Advisory Council on Alzheimer's Research, Care, and Services*. National Research Summit on Care, Services, and Supports for Persons with Dementia and Their Caregivers. Bethesda, MD: U.S. Department of Health and Human Services.

Hoffmann, T. C., P. P. Glasziou, I. Boutron, R. Milne, R. Perera, D. Moher, D. G. Altman, V. Barbour, H. Macdonald, M. Johnston, S. E. Lamb, M. Dixon-Woods, P. McCulloch, J. C. Wyatt, A.-W. Chan, and S. Michie. 2014. Better reporting of interventions: Template for intervention description and replication (TIDIER) checklist and guide. *BMJ* 348:g1687.

Houghton, C., K. Murphy, D. Brooker, and D. Casey. 2016. Healthcare staffs' experiences and perceptions of caring for people with dementia in the acute setting: Qualitative evidence synthesis. *International Journal of Nursing Studies* 61:104–116.

IOM (Institute of Medicine). 2000. *Promoting health: Intervention strategies from social and behavioral research*. Washington, DC: National Academy Press.

Jennings, L. A., A. Palimaru, M. G. Corona, X. E. Cagigas, K. D. Ramirez, T. Zhao, R. D. Hays, N. S. Wenger, and D. B. Reuben. 2017. Patient and caregiver goals for dementia care. *Quality of Life Research* 26(3):685–693.

Jennings, L. A., K. D. Ramirez, R. D. Hays, N. S. Wenger, and D. B. Reuben. 2018. Personalized goal attainment in dementia care: Measuring what persons with dementia and their caregivers want. *Journal of the American Geriatrics Society* 66(11):2120–2127.

Krauss, A. 2018. Why all randomised controlled trials produce biased results. *Annals of Medicine* 50(4):312–322.

Largent, E. A., and J. Karlawish. 2020. Rescuing research participants after Alzheimer trials stop early: Sending out an SOS. *JAMA Neurology* 77(4):413–414.

Lee, M., and S. Kolomer. 2005. Caregiver burden, dementia, and elder abuse in South Korea. *Journal of Elder Abuse & Neglect* 17(1):61–74.

Lewin, S., C. Glenton, H. Munthe-Kaas, B. Carlsen, C. J. Colvin, M. Gülmezoglu, J. Noyes, A. Booth, R. Garside, and A. Rashidian. 2015. Using qualitative evidence in decision making for health and social interventions: An approach to assess confidence in findings from qualitative evidence syntheses (GRADE-CERQual). *PLoS medicine* 12(10):e1001895.

Lewin, S., A. Booth, C. Glenton, H. Munthe-Kaas, A. Rashidian, M. Wainwright, M. A. Bohren, Ö. Tunçalp, C. J. Colvin, R. Garside, B. Carlsen, E. V. Langlois, and J. Noyes. 2018. Applying GRADE-CERQual to qualitative evidence synthesis findings: Introduction to the series. *Implementation Science* 13(1):2.

Liu-Seifert, H., S. W. Andersen, I. Lipkovich, K. C. Holdridge, and E. Siemers. 2015. A novel approach to delayed-start analyses for demonstrating disease-modifying effects in Alzheimer's disease. *PLoS One* 10(3):e0119632.

Livingston, G., J. Huntley, A. Sommerlad, D. Ames, C. Ballard, S. Banerjee, C. Brayne, A. Burns, J. Cohen-Mansfield, C. Cooper, S. G. Costafreda, A. Dias, N. Fox, L. N. Gitlin, R. Howard, H. C. Kales, M. Kivimäki, E. B. Larson, A. Ogunniyi, V. Orgeta, K. Ritchie, K. Rockwood, E. L. Sampson, Q. Samus, L. S. Schneider, G. Selbæk, L. Teri, and N. Mukadam. 2020a. Dementia prevention, intervention, and care: 2020 report of the Lancet Commission. *The Lancet* 396(10248):413–446.

Livingston, G., M. Manela, A. O'Keeffe, P. Rapaport, C. Cooper, M. Knapp, D. King, R. Romeo, Z. Walker, J. Hoe, C. Mummery, and J. Barber. 2020b. Clinical effectiveness of the start (strategies for relatives) psychological intervention for family carers and the effects on the cost of care for people with dementia: 6-year follow-up of a randomised controlled trial. *British Journal of Psychiatry* 216(1):35–42.

Lu, C. Y. 2009. Observational studies: A review of study designs, challenges and strategies to reduce confounding. *International Journal of Clinical Practice* 63(5):691–697.

Lykens, K., N. Moayad, S. Biswas, C. Reyes-Ortiz, and K. P. Singh. 2014. Impact of a community based implementation of REACH II program for caregivers of Alzheimer's patients. *PLoS One* 9(2):e89290.

Makaroun, L. K., R. L. Bachrach, and A.-M. Rosland. 2020. Elder abuse in the time of COVID-19-increased risks for older adults and their caregivers. *The American Journal of Geriatric Psychiatry* 28(8):876–880.

Mayeda, E. R., M. M. Glymour, C. P. Quesenberry, and R. A. Whitmer. 2016. Inequalities in dementia incidence between six racial and ethnic groups over 14 years. *Alzheimer's & Dementia* 12(3):216–224.

Mitchell, S. L., V. Mor, J. Harrison, and E. P. McCarthy. 2020. Embedded pragmatic trials in dementia care: Realizing the vision of the NIA IMPACT Collaboratory. *Journal of the American Geriatrics Society* 68(Suppl 2):S1–S7. https://doi.org/10.1111/jgs.16621.

Moberg, J., and M. Kramer. 2015. A brief history of the cluster randomised trial design. *Journal of the Royal Society of Medicine* 108(5):192–198.

Moberg, J., A. D. Oxman, S. Rosenbaum, H. J. Schünemann, G. Guyatt, S. Flottorp, C. Glenton, S. Lewin, A. Morelli, G. Rada, P. Alonso-Coello, E. Akl, M. Gulmezoglu, R. A. Mustafa, J. Singh, E. von Elm, J. Vogel, and J. Watine. 2018. The GRADE Evidence to Decision (EtD) framework for health system and public health decisions. *Health Research Policy and Systems* 16(1):45.

Morgan, D., M. Crossley, N. Stewart, A. Kirk, D. Forbes, C. D'Arcy, V. Dal Bello-Haas, L. McBain, M. O'Connell, J. Bracken, J. Kosteniuk, and A. Cammer. 2014. Evolution of a community-based participatory approach in a rural and remote dementia care research program. *Progress in Community Health Partnerships* 8(3):337–345.

Murray, E., S. Treweek, C. Pope, A. MacFarlane, L. Ballini, C. Dowrick, T. Finch, A. Kennedy, F. Mair, C. O'Donnell, B. N. Ong, T. Rapley, A. Rogers, and C. May. 2010. Normalisation process theory: A framework for developing, evaluating and implementing complex interventions. *BMC Medicine* 8(1):63.

NIA (National Institute on Aging). 2018. *Stage model for behavioral intervention development.* https://www.nia.nih.gov/research/dbsr/nih-stage-model-behavioral-intervention-development (accessed August 18, 2020).

NIA. n.d. *National strategy for recruitment and participation in Alzheimer's and related dementias clinical research.* https://www.nia.nih.gov/research/recruitment-strategy (accessed November 25, 2020).

NIH (National Institutes of Health). 2017a. *NIH policy on the dissemination of NIH-funded clinical trial information.* https://grants.nih.gov/policy/clinical-trials/reporting/understanding/nih-policy.htm (accessed August 12, 2020).

NIH. 2017b. *Requirements for registering & reporting NIH-funded clinical trials in clinicaltrials.Gov.* https://grants.nih.gov/policy/clinical-trials/reporting/index.htm (accessed December 11, 2020).

NORC at the University of Chicago. 2016. *Third annual report: HCIA disease-specific evaluation.* Bethesda, MD: NORC at the University of Chicago.

NQF (National Quality Forum). 2014. *Priority setting for healthcare performance measurement: Addressing performance measure gaps for dementia, including alzheimer's disease.* http://www.qualityforum.org/priority_setting_for_healthcare_performance_measurement_alzheimers_disease.aspx (accessed September 4, 2020).

Ofstedal, M. B., and D. R. Weir. 2011. Recruitment and retention of minority participants in the health and retirement study. *The Gerontologist* 51(Suppl 1):S8–S20. https://doi.org/10.1093/geront/gnq100.

Oh, S. S., J. Galanter, N. Thakur, M. Pino-Yanes, N. E. Barcelo, M. J. White, D. M. de Bruin, R. M. Greenblatt, K. Bibbins-Domingo, A. H. B. Wu, L. N. Borrell, C. Gunter, N. R. Powe, and E. G. Burchard. 2015. Diversity in clinical and biomedical research: A promise yet to be fulfilled. *PLoS Medicine* 12(12):e1001918.

Onken, L. S., K. M. Carroll, V. Shoham, B. N. Cuthbert, and M. Riddle. 2014. Reenvisioning clinical science: Unifying the discipline to improve the public health. *Clinical Psychological Science* 2(1):22–34.

Pawson, R., T. Greenhalgh, G. Harvey, and K. Walshe. 2005. Realist review—A new method of systematic review designed for complex policy interventions. *Journal of Health Services Research & Policy* 10(Suppl 1):21–34.

Phelan, J. C., and B. G. Link. 2015. Is racism a fundamental cause of inequalities in health? *Annual Review of Sociology* 41(1):311–330.

Pinquart, M., and S. Sörensen. 2011. Spouses, adult children, and children-in-law as caregivers of older adults: A meta-analytic comparison. *Psychology and Aging* 26(1):1–14.

Prince, M. J., A. Wimo, M. Guerchet, G. Ali, Y.-T. Wu , M. Prina, and Alzheimer's Disease International. 2015. *World Alzheimer report 2015: The global impact of dementia: An analysis of prevalence, incidence, cost and trends.* London, UK: Alzheimer's Disease International.

Proctor, E., H. Silmere, R. Raghavan, P. Hovmand, G. Aarons, A. Bunger, R. Griffey, and M. Hensley. 2011. Outcomes for implementation research: Conceptual distinctions, measurement challenges, and research agenda. *Administration and Policy in Mental Health* 38(2):65–76.

Quiñones, A. R., S. L. Mitchell, J. D. Jackson, M. P. Aranda, P. Dilworth-Anderson, E. P. McCarthy, and L. Hinton. 2020. Achieving health equity in embedded pragmatic trials for people living with dementia and their family caregivers. *Journal of the American Geriatrics Society* 68(S2):S8–S13.

Reilly, J. C., and C. Houghton. 2019. The experiences and perceptions of care in acute settings for patients living with dementia: A qualitative evidence synthesis. *International Journal of Nursing Studies* 96:82–90.

Rencher, W. C., and L. E. Wolf. 2013. Redressing past wrongs: Changing the common rule to increase minority voices in research. *American Journal of Public Health* 103(12):2136–2140.

Richiardi, L., R. Bellocco, and D. Zugna. 2013. Mediation analysis in epidemiology: Methods, interpretation and bias. *International Journal of Epidemiology* 42(5):1511–1519.

Sayer, C. 2016. "Time spent at home"—A patient-defined outcome. *NEJM Catalyst* 2(2).

Sim, J. 2019. Should treatment effects be estimated in pilot and feasibility studies? *Pilot and Feasibility Studies* 5(1):107.

Skinner, J. S., N. A. Williams, A. Richmond, J. Brown, A. H. Strelnick, K. Calhoun, E. H. De Loney, S. Allen, A. Pirie, and C. H. Wilkins. 2018. Community experiences and perceptions of clinical and translational research and researchers. *Progress in Community Health Partnerships* 12(3):263–271.

Smith, A. S., and E. Trevelyan. 2019. *The older population in rural America: 2012–2016.* Washington, DC: U.S. Census Bureau.

Steenland, K., F. C. Goldstein, A. Levey, and W. Wharton. 2016. A meta-analysis of Alzheimer's disease incidence and prevalence comparing African-Americans and Caucasians. *Journal of Alzheimer's Disease* 50(1):71–76.

Tobe, S. W., M. Moy Lum-Kwong, S. Von Sychowski, K. Kandukur, A. Kiss, and V. Flintoft. 2014. Hypertension management initiative prospective cohort study: Comparison between immediate and delayed intervention groups. *Journal of Human Hypertension* 28(1):44–50.

U.S. Census Bureau. 2012. *U.S. Census Bureau projections show a slower growing, older, more diverse nation a half century from now.* https://www.census.gov/newsroom/releases/archives/population/cb12-243.html (accessed August 12, 2020).

U.S. Census Bureau. 2020. *National population by characteristics: 2010–2019.* https://www.census.gov/data/tables/time-series/demo/popest/2010s-national-detail.html (accessed August 10, 2020).

Vernooij-Dassen, M., and E. Moniz-Cook. 2014. Raising the standard of applied dementia care research: Addressing the implementation error. *Aging & Mental Health* 18(7):809–814.

Viswanathan, M., A. Ammerman, E. Eng, G. Garlehner, K. N. Lohr, D. Griffith, S. Rhodes, C. Samuel-Hodge, S. Maty, and L. Lux. 2004. Community based participatory research: Assessing the evidence: Summary. In *AHRQ evidence report summaries.* Agency for Healthcare Research and Quality (US).

Wang, B., D. R. Hoover, T. Beck, and X. Dong. 2020. A vulnerability risk index of self-neglect in a community-dwelling older population. *Journal of the American Geriatrics Society* 68(4):809–816.

Weiner, M. F., K. Martin-Cook, D. A. Svetlik, K. Saine, B. Foster, and C. S. Fontaine. 2000. The quality of life in late-stage dementia (QUALID) scale. *Journal of the American Medical Directors Association* 1(3):114–116.

Wells, K., and L. Jones. 2009. "Research" in community-partnered, participatory research. *Journal of the American Medical Association* 302(3):320–321.

Wharton, T. C., and B. K. Ford. 2014. What is known about dementia care recipient violence and aggression against caregivers? *Journal of Gerontological Social Work* 57(5):460–477.

Wiegersma, P. A., A. Hofman, and G. A. Zielhuis. 2001. Evaluation of community-wide interventions: The ecologic case-referent study design. *European Journal of Epidemiology* 17(6):551–557.

Wiglesworth, A., L. Mosqueda, R. Mulnard, S. Liao, L. Gibbs, and W. Fitzgerald. 2010. Screening for abuse and neglect of people with dementia. *Journal of the American Geriatrics Society* 58(3):493–500.

Williams, I. C., and G. Corbie-Smith. 2006. Investigator beliefs and reported success in recruiting minority participants. *Contemporary Clinical Trials* 27(6):580–586.

Yan, E., and T. Kwok. 2011. Abuse of older Chinese with dementia by family caregivers: An inquiry into the role of caregiver burden. *International Journal of Geriatric Psychiatry* 26(5):527–535.

APPENDIX A

AGENCY FOR HEALTHCARE RESEARCH AND QUALITY SYSTEMATIC REVIEW AND INCLUSION CRITERIA

The Agency for Healthcare Research and Quality (AHRQ) systematic review *Care Interventions for People Living with Dementia and Their Caregivers*, which provided the primary evidence base for this study, can be found here: https://effectivehealthcare.ahrq.gov/products/care-interventions-pwd/report (accessed January 29, 2021). Table A-1 presents the inclusion criteria applied by the systematic review authors.

TABLE A-1 PICOTS Inclusion Criteria for AHRQ Systematic Review

Element	PLWD	PLWD Caregiver
Population	**PLWD,** including individuals with possible or diagnosed AD/ADRD PLWD Subgroups: Age, sex, sexual orientation/gender identity, race/ethnicity, education, socioeconomic status, prior disability, age at diagnosis, dementia type, dementia severity (e.g., stage of dementia [early stage, moderate, or severe], level of cognitive impairment rate of cognitive decline), family/household characteristics, health insurance, geographic location (e.g., urban, rural), setting type	**Informal PLWD Caregivers,** such as spouses, family, friends, and volunteers Informal PLWD Caregiver Subgroups, including age, sex, sexual orientation/gender identity, race/ethnicity, family history of dementia, education, socioeconomic status, employment status, relationship with PLWD, living distance from PLWD, dementia care training, general health status, caregiving networks, setting type **Formal PLWD Caregivers,** such as certified nursing assistants (CNAs), home health aides, auxiliary workers, personal care aides, hospice aides, promotoras or promotores, and community health workers Formal PLWD Caregiver Subgroups, including age, sex, race/ethnicity, education, job position, skill, training, general health status, setting type

TABLE A-1 Continued

Element	PLWD	PLWD Caregiver
Intervention	Any nondrug care intervention intended to benefit PLWD **except** interventions to treat conditions other than dementia, including but not limited to CPAP, and those that use supplements/natural products	Any care intervention intended to support informal PLWD caregivers' well-being **except** interventions to treat health conditions unrelated to providing care to PLWD Any care intervention intended to support formal PLWD caregivers' well-being except interventions to treat health conditions unrelated to providing care to PLWD Any care delivery intervention to improve how care is delivered if the training intervention is incorporated as on-going operational procedures into the structure or processes of the organization. Interventions carried out by higher education organizations or professional organizations to provide training toward licensed professionals, and continuing education for degreed health professionals are also excluded
Comparator	Inactive Comparator: No intervention, usual care, waitlist, attention control Active Comparator: Different intervention	Inactive Comparator: No intervention, usual care, waitlist, attention control Active Comparator: Different intervention

continued

TABLE A-1 Continued

Element	PLWD	PLWD Caregiver
Outcomes	Quality of life and subjective well-being Burden of care Satisfaction with care Perceived support Expenditures/financial burden (informal caregivers) Health-related outcomes: Psychological health (e.g., depression, anxiety) Neuropsychiatric symptoms (including apathy, aggression, and agitation) Function (e.g., ADL, IADL, ability to care for one's self, ability to recreate/socialize) Weight loss Sleep problems Use of restraints Use of anti-psychotics Harm reduction (e.g., driving, firearms) Palliative care/hospice outcomes: Completion of advanced directives Comfort during dying process Concordance with preferred location of death Social/Community level outcomes: Engagement in community activities Perceived inclusion Safety/perceived safety Utilization of health care service outcomes: Admission to nursing home Access to care and services ICU and ED usage Hospital admission and readmission Primary, Specialty, Long-term Care usage Quality of care and services (e.g., overutilization of unnecessary antibiotics, other quality care metrics)	Quality of life and subjective well-being Burden of care Satisfaction with care for PLWD (informal caregivers) Perceived support Expenditures/financial burden (informal caregivers) Health-related outcomes: Psychological health (e.g., depression, anxiety) Immune function (e.g., inflammation or cortisol) Sleep problems Weight loss due to stress Health behaviors (e.g., exercise, substance use) Caregiving self-efficacy Confidence to manage caregiver tasks Social/community-level outcomes (informal caregivers): Engagement in community activities Perceived inclusion Safety/perceived safety Turnover and retention (formal caregivers) Utilization of health care service (e.g., physician visits, antidepressant or antianxiety medication usage) Societal costs including caregiving time/time spent on activities Harms, including isolation, loneliness, perceived stigma, caregiver PTSD

TABLE A-1 Continued

Element	PLWD	PLWD Caregiver
Outcomes (continued)	Societal costs, including caregiving time/time spent on activities Harms, including isolation, loneliness, perceived stigma, suicidal ideation or suicide, elder abuse (e.g., physical harm, abuse, neglect, exploitation, family violence)	
Timing	No minimum duration or follow-up	No minimum duration or follow-up
Setting	Any setting; no exclusion based on geographic location or setting. Includes home, home health care, adult day care, acute care settings, social service agencies, nursing homes, assisted living, memory care units, hospice, rehabilitation centers/skilled nursing facilities, long-distance caregiving, and nonplace-based settings	Any setting; no exclusion based on geographic locations or setting. Includes home, home health care, adult day care, acute care settings, social service agencies, nursing homes, assisted living, memory care units, hospice, rehabilitation centers/skilled nursing facilities, long-distance caregiving, and nonplace-based settings

NOTE: ADL = activity of daily living; CPAP = continuous positive airway pressure; ED = emergency department; IADL = instrumental activity of daily living; ICU = intensive care unit; PLWD = person living with dementia; PTSD = posttraumatic stress disorder.
SOURCE: Excerpted from Butler et al., 2020; for additional details, see Appendix A of Butler et al., 2020.

REFERENCE

Butler, M., J. E. Gaugler, K. M. C. Talley, H. I. Abdi, P. J. Desai, S. Duval, M. L. Forte, V. A. Nelson, W. Ng, J. M. Ouellette, E. Ratner, J. Saha, T. Shippee, B. L. Wagner, T. J. Wilt, and L. Yeshi. 2020. Care interventions for people living with dementia and their caregivers. *Comparative Effectiveness Review No. 231*. Rockville, MD: Agency for Healthcare Research and Quality. doi: 10.23970/AHRQEPCCER231.

APPENDIX B

PUBLIC MEETING AGENDAS

Open Sessions: November 12–13, 2018

DAY ONE—MONDAY, NOVEMBER 12

10:45 am **Welcome and Introductions**
Eric Larson, Kaiser Permanente Washington Health Research Institute, Committee Chair

10:50 am **Delivery of Study Charge and Initial Discussion**
Objectives:
- Receive study background and charge from the National Institute on Aging (NIA), discuss task with the sponsor, and determine scope of committee's work.
- Receive an overview of the Agency for Healthcare Research and Quality (AHRQ) process for systematic reviews.
- Receive an update from the Evidence-based Practice Center (EPC) on progress to date and questions for the committee.
- Clarify issues identified by the committee and seek answers to questions.
- Discuss report audience.

Delivery of Charge
Richard Hodes, Director, NIA (10 minutes)

Overview of AHRQ Process
Kim Wittenberg, Health Scientist Administrator, AHRQ (5 minutes, by webcast)

Overview of EPC Progress to Date and Areas for Committee Input
Mary Butler and Joseph Gaugler, Minnesota Evidence-based Practice Center (15 minutes)

Discussion About Committee Charge and Process (30 minutes)
Speakers above, plus additional discussants from NIA:
Marie A. Bernard, Deputy Director
John Haaga, Director, Division of Behavioral and Social Research
Elena Fazio, Health Scientist Administrator, Division of Behavioral and Social Research
Melinda Kelley, Director, Office of Legislation, Policy, and International Activities

11:50 am **Lunch**

12:45 pm **Key Themes from the 2017 *National Research Summit on Care, Services, and Supports for Persons with Dementia and Their Caregivers***
Laura Gitlin, Dean, College of Nursing and Health Professions, Drexel University

1:00 pm **Perspective of a Person Living with Dementia**
Mary Radnofsky, Dementia rights advocate

1:15 pm **Discussion About the Systematic Review Key Questions and Scope**
Objective: Discussion among NIA, EPC, and the committee about the draft systematic review key questions and scope, and about the EPC's questions for the committee.
Richard Hodes, Marie A. Bernard, John Haaga, Elena Fazio, and Melinda Kelley, NIA
Mary Butler and Joseph Gaugler, Minnesota EPC

3:00 pm	**Public Comment Period** Members of the public who register will have 3 minutes to comment on any topic related to the study charge.
3:15 pm	**Adjourn Day One Open Session**

DAY TWO—TUESDAY, NOVEMBER 13

10:00 am	**Introductory Remarks** *Eric Larson,* Committee Chair
10:05 am	**Continued Discussion About the Systematic Review Key Questions and Scope** *Objective:* Discuss any remaining issues, questions, or points of clarification related to the draft systematic review key questions and scope. *Richard Hodes, Marie A. Bernard, John Haaga, Elena Fazio, and Melinda Kelley,* NIA *Mary Butler and Joseph Gaugler,* Minnesota EPC
11:30 am	**Adjourn Day Two Open Session**

Open Session: February 4, 2019

4:00 pm	**Welcome and Opening Remarks** *Eric Larson,* Committee Chair
4:05 pm	**Overview of EPC Draft Protocol and Questions for the Committee** *Mary Butler* and *Joseph Gaugler,* Minnesota EPC
4:15 pm	**Discussion** moderated by *Eric Larson,* Committee Chair
6:00 pm	**Adjourn**

Public Workshop: April 15, 2020

SESSION 1: INTRODUCTION, STUDY CHARGE, AND DRAFT SYSTEMATIC REVIEW

Session Objectives:

- Receive a briefing from the study sponsor on the committee's charge.
- Receive an overview of the draft AHRQ/EPC systematic review.
- Discuss care interventions and outcomes that are of most interest to people living with dementia and their caregivers.

10:00 am **Welcome and Overview of Workshop Objectives**
Eric Larson, Kaiser Permanente Washington Health Research Institute, Committee Chair

10:10 am **Background and Overview of the Committee's Charge**
Richard Hodes, NIA

10:25 am **Overview of the Draft AHRQ/EPC Systematic Review**
Mary Butler, Minnesota EPC
Joseph Gaugler, Minnesota EPC

10:45 am **Discussion with Committee Members**

11:30 am **Perspectives from a Caregiver: What Care Interventions and Outcomes Are Most Important?**
Janet Michel, family caregiver

11:40 am **Discussion with Committee Members**

11:50 am **Lunch**

SESSION 2: PERSPECTIVES ON "READINESS FOR DISSEMINATION AND IMPLEMENTATION"

Session Objectives:
NIA has asked the National Academies committee to make recommendations regarding which care interventions for individuals with dementia and their caregivers are "ready for dissemination and implementation on a broad scale." To explore this concept in the specific context of the draft AHRQ/EPC systematic review, this session will engage stakeholders and decision

makers from advocacy organizations, associations, foundations, care systems, and implementation science to:

- Discuss what "ready for dissemination and implementation on a broad scale" means. How should this be assessed? What kinds of evidence do different stakeholders and decision makers look for?
- Provide input on the AHRQ/EPC draft systematic review.

12:30 pm	**Session Objectives** *Jason Karlawish,* University of Pennsylvania, committee member and session moderator
12:35 pm	**Panel 1: Perspectives from Advocacy Organizations and Associations** *Moderated discussion with:* *Lynn Feinberg,* AARP *Kathleen Kelly,* Family Caregiving Alliance *Douglas Pace,* Alzheimer's Association
1:10 pm	**Discussion with Committee Members**
1:30 pm	**Panel II: Perspectives from Care Systems and Payers** *Moderated discussion with:* *Patrick Courneya,* HealthPartners *David Gifford,* American Health Care Association *Shari Ling,* Centers for Medicare & Medicaid Services *Lewis Sandy,* UnitedHealth Group
2:10 pm	**Discussion with Committee Members**
2:30 pm	**Panel III: Perspectives from Implementation Science** *Moderated discussion with:* *Laura Gitlin,* Drexel University *Melissa Simon,* Northwestern University
3:00 pm	**Discussion with Committee Members**
3:20 pm	**Break**

SESSION 3: STATE OF THE EVIDENCE AND METHODOLOGICAL CONSIDERATIONS

Session Objectives:

- Continue to reflect on the draft AHRQ/EPC systematic review results, explore the current state of evidence, and discuss which care interventions for individuals with dementia and their caregivers may be ready for dissemination and implementation on a broad scale.
    - Particular focus will be given to racial, ethnic, cultural, language, and socioeconomic considerations, across all aspects of the systematic review results.
- Discuss emerging data on care interventions that did not meet the evidentiary standard of the systematic review and data expected from studies under way that were not published in time for inclusion in the systematic review, and identify gaps and areas for future research.

3:30 pm **Session Objectives**
XinQi Dong, Rutgers University, committee member and session moderator

3:35 pm **Interventions for People with Dementia**
Linda Teri, University of Washington

3:45 pm **Interventions for Caregivers and Care Delivery Interventions**
Richard Schulz, University of Pittsburgh

3:55 pm **Cultural Modifications**
J. Neil Henderson, University of Minnesota

4:05 pm **Methodological Considerations and Treatment of Non-RCT Data**
Jennifer Weuve, Boston University

4:15 pm **Discussion Among Speakers and Committee Members**

4:50 pm **Closing Remarks**
Eric Larson, Committee Chair

5:00 pm **Public Session Adjourns**

Open Session: May 29, 2020

Open session objective: A group of people living with dementia and caregivers will provide perspectives on the draft AHRQ/EPC systematic review and input into the National Academies committee's report.

Discussion questions:

- What would you like the National Academies committee to consider in drafting its report?
- The draft AHRQ/EPC systematic review identified two interventions as supported by low strength evidence (see background information below):
  - How important to you are the outcomes targeted by these two interventions?
  - Based on the brief descriptions below, would you be inclined to seek out these two interventions, and would you welcome them if they were offered to you?

2:30 pm **Welcome**
Eric Larson, Committee Chair

2:35 pm **Opening Remarks on the Questions Above (~3 minutes each)**
Cynthia Huling Hummel, living with dementia, Elmira, New York
Karen Love, Dementia Action Alliance
Maria Martinez Israelite, care partner, Washington, DC
John Richard (JR) Pagan, living with dementia, Woodbridge, Virginia
Brian Van Buren, living with dementia, Charlotte, North Carolina
Geraldine Woolfolk, care partner, Oakland, California

3:00 pm **Discussion with Committee Members**

3:15 pm **Adjourn Open Session**

Open Session: September 16, 2020

Open meeting objective: Receive an overview from the Minnesota EPC about changes from the draft to the final AHRQ systematic review.

11:00 am	**Welcome and Meeting Objectives** *Eric Larson,* Kaiser Permanente Washington Health Research Institute, Committee Chair
11:05 am	**Overview of Changes from the Draft to the Final AHRQ Systematic Review** *Mary Butler,* Minnesota EPC *Joseph Gaugler,* Minnesota EPC
11:20 am	**Discussion with Committee Members**
12:00 pm	**Adjourn Open Session**

APPENDIX C

BIOGRAPHICAL SKETCHES OF COMMITTEE MEMBERS AND STAFF

COMMITTEE MEMBERS

Eric B. Larson, M.D., M.P.H. (*Chair*), is a senior investigator at the Kaiser Permanente Washington Health Research Institute, the former vice president for research and health care innovation for Kaiser Permanente Washington, and the executive director of the Institute. A graduate of Harvard Medical School, Dr. Larson trained in internal medicine at Beth Israel Hospital in Boston, completed a Robert Wood Johnson Clinical Scholars and M.P.H. at the University of Washington (UW), and then served as the chief resident of University Hospital in Seattle. He served as the medical director of the UW Medical Center and the associate dean for clinical affairs from 1989 to 2002 and remains a clinical professor of medicine and health services at UW. His research spans a range of general medicine topics and has focused on aging and dementia, including a long-running study of aging and cognitive change set in Kaiser Permanente Washington, formerly Group Health Cooperative—The UW/Group Health Alzheimer's Disease Patient Registry/Adult Changes in Thought Study. Dr. Larson has served as the president of the Society of General Internal Medicine, the chair of the Office of Technology Assessment/U.S. Department of Health and Human Services Advisory Panel on Alzheimer's Disease and Related Disorders, and was the chair of the board of regents (2004–2005) of the American College of Physicians. He is an elected member of the National Academy of Medicine.

Marilyn Albert, Ph.D., is the director of the Division of Cognitive Neuroscience, a professor of neurology at the Johns Hopkins University School of Medicine, and the director of the Johns Hopkins Alzheimer's Disease Research Center. She received her Ph.D. in physiological psychology from McGill University in Montreal and completed a fellowship in neuropsychology at the Boston University School of Medicine. She served on the faculty of the Harvard Medical School from 1981 to 2003. She moved to Johns Hopkins in 2003. Dr. Albert focuses on the cognitive and brain changes associated with aging and Alzheimer's disease (AD). Her work has delineated the cognitive changes associated with aging and early AD. She has also identified lifestyle factors that promote maintenance of mental abilities with advancing age. Dr. Albert's research currently focuses on the early identification of AD and potential ways of monitoring the progression of disease to permit early intervention.

María P. Aranda, Ph.D., M.S.W., M.P.A., is an associate professor at the University of Southern California (USC) Suzanne Dworak-Peck School of Social Work and the executive director of the USC Edward R. Roybal Institute on Aging. She leads the Outreach, Recruitment and Engagement Core of the USC Alzheimer's Disease Research Center. Dr. Aranda's research, teaching, and practice interests address the study of psychosocial care of adult and late-life psychiatric and neurocognitive disorders, including depression and Alzheimer's disease and related dementias. She examines racial and ethnic diversity in the delivery of health and mental health services, disparities in health and health care, and testing of psychosocial interventions to alleviate illness burden among persons living with medical and psychiatric illnesses and their family care partners. Dr. Aranda has served as the principal investigator or the co-investigator on several key studies funded by and/or in collaboration with the National Institute of Mental Health, the National Cancer Institute, the Patient-Centered Outcomes Research Institute, the State of California Alzheimer's Disease Program, The John A. Hartford Foundation/Gerontological Society of America, the California Community Foundation, the National Institute of Rehabilitation and Research, the Alzheimer's Association/Health Resources and Services Administration, the Los Angeles County Department of Mental Health, and the Larson Endowment for Innovative Research.

She co-pioneered a state-of-the-art family support program ("El Portal") for low-income, Spanish-speaking families dealing with neurodegenerative disorders, which is a national model for family caregiving in hard-to-reach communities. Dr. Aranda has served on several consensus study committees of the National Academies of Sciences, Engineering, and Medicine, including on the geriatric workforce in mental health and substance use service sectors, family caregiving to older adults with functional limitations, and financial capacity determination among Social Security beneficiaries.

Christopher M. Callahan, M.D., MACP, is a professor of medicine at the Indiana University School of Medicine. He also serves as the chief research and development officer at Eskenazi Health, one of the nation's largest safety net health systems. He is an active research scientist in the Indiana University Center for Aging Research at the Regenstrief Institute. His research seeks to improve outcomes for older adults with late-life depression and dementia, focused on innovative models of care that support generalist physicians in their day-to-day provision of health to older adults. Dr. Callahan has spent more than two decades developing and exploring new treatment models for older adults and was recognized in 2016 with the Edward Henderson Award from the American Geriatrics Society. He continues to provide care for older adults in the Sandra Eskenazi Center for Brain Care Innovation. Dr. Callahan attended the St. Louis University School of Medicine, completed his internship and residency at Baylor College of Medicine, and fellowship at the Indiana University School of Medicine.

Eileen M. Crimmins, Ph.D., is the AARP professor of gerontology in the Leonard Davis School of Gerontology at the University of Southern California (USC). She is a member of the National Academy of Sciences and the National Academy of Medicine, a fellow of the American Association for the Advancement of Science, and is currently the director of the USC/University of California, Los Angeles, Center on Biodemography and Population Health, one of the Demography of Aging Centers supported by the National Institute on Aging (NIA). She is also the director of the Multidisciplinary Training in Gerontology Program and the NIA-sponsored Network on Biological Risk. Dr. Crimmins is a co-investigator of the Health and Retirement Study in the United States. Much of Dr. Crimmins's research has focused on changes over time in health and mortality. Dr. Crimmins has been instrumental in organizing and promoting the recent integration of the measurement of biological indicators in large population surveys. She served as the co-chair of a committee for the National Academies of Sciences, Engineering, and Medicine to address why life expectancy in the United States is falling so far behind that of other countries. She has also co-edited several books with a focus on international aging, mortality, and health expectancy: *Determining Health Expectancies*; *Longer Life and Healthy Aging*; *Human Longevity, Individual Life Duration, and the Growth of the Oldest-Old Population*; *International Handbook of Adult Mortality*; *Explaining Diverging Levels of Longevity in High-Income Countries*; and *International Differences in Mortality at Older Ages: Dimensions and Sources*. She has received the Kleemeier Award for Research from the Gerontological Society of America.

Peggye Dilworth-Anderson, Ph.D., is a professor of health policy and management at the Gillings School of Global Public Health at the University of North Carolina (UNC) at Chapel Hill. Her research focus is on health disparities and Alzheimer's disease (AD) with an emphasis on building knowledge for the scientific and lay communities to inform conducting culturally relevant research and disseminating information about AD and related disorders in medically underserved diverse populations. In recognition of her research in aging, Dr. Dilworth-Anderson received the Pearmain Prize for Excellence in Research on Aging from the University of Southern California (USC) Edward R. Roybal Institute on Aging. UNC awarded her the University Diversity Award in recognition of her commitment to diversity and inclusion in research, teaching, and leadership. She received the Ronald and Nancy Reagan Alzheimer's Research Award for her research contributions on AD in medically underserved populations from the Alzheimer's Association. Dr. Dilworth-Anderson has served in numerous leadership roles, some of which include the president of the Gerontological Society of America; a member of the Global Council on Brain Health, committees of the National Academies of Sciences, Engineering, and Medicine; the National Alzheimer's Association Medical and Scientific Council; the Board of Directors of the National Alzheimer's Association and Eastern North Carolina Chapter; the National Research Advisory Council of the Institute on Aging/National Institutes of Health.

XinQi Dong, M.D., M.P.H., is the director of the Institute for Health, Health Care Policy, and Aging Research at Rutgers University as well as the inaugural Henry Rutgers professor of population health sciences. Dr. Dong has published extensively on the topics of violence prevention in global populations with more than 260 peer-reviewed publications and is leading a longitudinal epidemiological study (The PINE Study) of 3,300 Chinese older adults to quantify relationships among culture, violence, and health outcomes. Dr. Dong is the principal investigator of eight federally funded grants and also has mentored many trainees and faculties to success. He is the principal investigator of the National Institute on Aging (NIA)-funded Resource Centers for Minority Aging Research. Dr. Dong served on many editorial boards, was the guest editor-in-chief for the *Journal of Aging Health* and the *Journal of Gerontology: Medical Sciences*, and edited the key textbook on elder abuse—the field's largest collection of research, practice, and policy.

Dr. Dong was the recipient of the Paul Beeson Award by NIA, the National Physician Advocacy Merit Award by the Institute for Medicine as a Profession, the Nobuo Maeda International Aging and Public Health Research Award by the American Public Health Association (APHA), the National Award for Excellence by APHA, the Maxwell Pollack Award in Productive Aging, the Joseph Freeman Award, and the Powell Lawton Award by the Gerontological Society of America. He was also awarded the Rosalie Wolf Award by the National Committee on the Prevention of Elder Abuse and the Outstanding Scientific Achievement for Clinical Investigation Award by the American Geriatric Society. Dr. Dong was elected to be a commissioner for the Commission on Law and Aging of the American Bar Association. In 2017, Dr. Dong received the Edward Busse Award by the International Congress of Gerontology and Geriatrics.

Dr. Dong has been a strong advocate for advancing population health issues in underrepresented communities across the local, national, and international levels. Internationally, Dr. Dong has worked with multiple institutions in China as well as the Chinese National Committee on Aging to further dialogue between the United States and China collaborative on elder justice and mental health. Dr. Dong served as a senior advisor for the U.S. Department of Health and Human Services under the Obama administration. His policy and advocacy work with the U.S. Department of Justice and the Centers for Disease Control and Prevention have also shaped the national agenda on the surveillance and preventive strategies combating the issues of violence prevention. In 2011, Dr. Dong was appointed as a member of the National Academies of Sciences, Engineering, and Medicine's Forum on Global Violence Prevention. Subsequently, he chaired the workshop on elder abuse prevention. In 2017, Dr. Dong was invited to be the planning committee member for the Board on Global Health to chart the future of violence prevention effort at the National Academies. In 2018, Dr. Dong was elected to the American Society of Clinical Investigation and was awarded the Health Equity Award from the Robert Wood Johnson Foundation.

An immigrant to the United States, Dr. Dong grew up in a rural village near Nanjing, China. He received his B.A. in biology and economics from the University of Chicago, his M.D. at Rush University College of Medicine, and his M.P.H. in epidemiology at the University of Illinois at Chicago. He completed his internal medicine residency and geriatric fellowship at the Yale University Medical Center.

Miguel Hernán, M.D., Dr.P.H., conducts research to learn what works to improve human health. Together with his collaborators, he designs analyses of health care databases, epidemiologic studies, and randomized trials. Dr. Hernán teaches clinical data science at the Harvard Medical School; clinical epidemiology at the Harvard-Massachusetts Institute of Technology Division of Health Sciences and Technology; and causal inference methodology at the Harvard T.H. Chan School of Public Health, where he is the Kolokotrones professor of biostatistics and epidemiology. His edX course Causal Diagrams and his book *Causal Inference*, co-authored with

James Robins, are freely available online and widely used for the training of researchers. Dr. Hernán is an elected fellow of the American Association for the Advancement of Science and of the American Statistical Association; an editor of *Epidemiology*; and the past or current associate editor of *Biometrics*, the *American Journal of Epidemiology*, and the *Journal of the American Statistical Association.*

Ronald Hickman, Jr., Ph.D., RN, ACNP-BC, FNAP, FAAN, is the Ruth M. Anderson Endowed professor and the associate dean for research at the Frances Payne Bolton School of Nursing at Case Western Reserve University. Dr. Hickman's research integrates knowledge from several disciplinary domains to understand psychosocial and biological mechanisms that influence how persons with cognitive impairment and their family caregivers make health-related decisions and provide technology-based decision support.

Helen Hovdesven, M.A., holds an M.A. in health advocacy from Sarah Lawrence College. Prior to retiring, Ms. Hovdesven was a patient representative and acting director of patient relations at a tertiary care facility. She was involved with direct patient care, helping patients and their families navigate the health care system, ensuring their medical and health care needs and collaborating with other health care providers to mediate conflicts and facilitate change. She was also an HIV counselor, organ donor requestor, and volunteer trainer and coordinator for Reach to Recovery. Ms. Hovdesven also served on the Ethics Committee and Child Protection Services Committee. Ms. Hovdesven is currently the co-chair of the Patient Family Advisory Council (PFAC) at the Johns Hopkins Memory and Alzheimer's Treatment Center, and has been involved with PFAC since its launch in 2008 and served as the chair for more than 7 years. She is also involved with the Johns Hopkins Brain Autopsy Program and has been an advisory board member of the Department of Psychiatry and Behavioral Sciences since 2003. Ms. Hovdesven is dedicated to Alzheimer's research, including the needs of caregivers, having been a caregiver for her late husband, Arne. She has also completed a series of podcasts for Johns Hopkins, "Alzheimer's from Diagnosis to Death" and "Brain Autopsy," sharing their personal story.

Rebecca A. Hubbard, Ph.D., is an associate professor of biostatistics in the Department of Biostatistics, Epidemiology, and Informatics at the University of Pennsylvania Perelman School of Medicine. Dr. Hubbard's research focuses on the development and application of statistical methodology for observational studies using real-world data, including electronic health records and administrative claims. This work encompasses the evaluation of screening and diagnostic test performance, methods for comparative effectiveness studies, and health services research. Dr. Hubbard's methodological research has been applied to studies of cancer epidemiology, aging and dementia, pharmacoepidemiology, women's health, and behavioral health. Dr. Hubbard received a B.S. (ecology and evolution, summa cum laude) from the University of Pittsburgh, an M.Sc. (epidemiology) from the University of Edinburgh, an M.Sc. (applied statistics, with Honors) from Oxford University, and a Ph.D. (biostatistics) from the University of Washington.

Jason Karlawish, M.D., is a professor of medicine, medical ethics, health policy, and neurology at the University of Pennsylvania and cares for patients at the Penn Memory Center, which he co-directs. His research focuses on issues at the intersections of bioethics, aging, and the neurosciences. He leads the Penn Program for Precision Medicine for the Brain (P3MB). P3MB developed standards for Alzheimer's disease (AD) biomarker disclosure and investigates the clinical impacts of this knowledge on persons with AD and their families. He has investigated the development and translation of AD treatments and biomarker-based diagnostics, informed consent, quality of life, research and treatment decision making, and voting by persons with cognitive impairment and residents of long-term care facilities. Dr. Karlawish has disseminated his research in leading textbooks of medicine and bioethics, testimony to the Senate Select Committee on Aging, and the U.S. Department of Health and Human Services Subcommittee on the Inclusion of Individuals with Impaired Decision-making in Research, and collaborations with the Alzheimer's Disease Cooperative Study, the Alzheimer's Association, the American Bar Association's Commission on Law and Aging, AARP's Global Council on Brain Health, the U.S. Department of Housing and Urban Development, the National Academy of Medicine (he served on the National Academies of Sciences, Engineering, and Medicine's committee to address the public health challenges of cognitive aging), the State of Vermont, the U.S. Election Assistance Commission, and the U.S. Government Accountability Office. He is an international proponent of mobile polling, a method of bringing the vote to long-term care facilities that minimizes fraud and maximizes voter rights. In a widely publicized essay in the *Journal of the American Medical Association*, he introduced the concept of "desktop medicine," a theory of medicine that recognizes how risk and its numerical representations are transforming medicine, medical care, and health. He studied medicine at Northwestern University and trained in internal medicine and geriatric medicine at the Johns Hopkins University and the University of Chicago.

Robyn I. Stone, Dr.P.H., is the senior vice president for research at LeadingAge and the co-director of the LeadingAge LTSS Center @UMass

Boston. She is a noted researcher and an internationally recognized authority on long-term care and aging policy and has held senior research and policy development, program evaluation, large-scale demonstrations and other applied research activities in those areas for more than 40 years. Dr. Stone has held senior research and policy positions in both the federal government and the private sector, including serving in the U.S. Department of Health and Human Services as deputy assistant secretary for disability, aging, and long-term care policy and as the assistant secretary for aging in the Clinton administration. Her work bridges the worlds of research, policy, and practice to improve the care delivered to older adults—particularly lower-income populations—and to ensure the best quality of life for these individuals and their families. Dr. Stone is a distinguished speaker and has been published widely in the areas of long-term care policy and quality, chronic care for older adults and people with disabilities, aging services workforce development, the link between low-income senior housing and health, and family caregiving. She is a fellow of the Gerontological Society of America and the National Academy of Social Insurance and was elected to the National Academy of Medicine in 2014. She serves on numerous provider and nonprofit boards that focus on aging issues.

Jennifer L. Wolff, Ph.D., is the Eugene and Mildred Lipitz professor and the director of the Roger C. Lipitz Center for Integrated Health Care. She is an expert and thought leader in research and policy relating to the care of persons with complex health needs and disabilities. She has made major contributions to increasing understanding of the role of family caregivers in the interactions of older adults with the medical community. She has been involved in the development and evaluation of numerous initiatives aimed at better supporting older adults and their family caregivers, including applied research to develop practical tools and strategies that may be readily deployed in care delivery. Her research has been published in a wide range of journals, including the *New England Journal of Medicine*, the *Journal of the American Medical Association*, the *Journal of the American Geriatrics Society*, *Social Science and Medicine*, and *Health Affairs*. She has led projects that have been funded by the National Institute on Aging, the National Institute of Mental Health, AARP, the Jacob and Valeria Langeloth Foundation, the Milbank Memorial Fund, and Atlantic Philanthropies. Dr. Wolff directs the Roger C. Lipitz Center for Integrated Health Care and is a core member of the Center for Health Services and Outcomes Research, the Center on Aging and Health, and the Center on Innovative Care in Aging. She holds a joint appointment in the Johns Hopkins University School of Medicine's Division of Geriatric Medicine and Gerontology.

STAFF

Clare Stroud, Ph.D. (*Study Director*), is a senior program officer with the National Academies of Sciences, Engineering, and Medicine. In this capacity, she serves as the director for the Committee on Care Interventions for Individuals with Dementia and Their Caregivers. She also serves as the director of the Forum on Neuroscience and Nervous System Disorders, which brings together leaders from government, academia, industry, and nonprofit organizations to discuss key challenges and emerging issues in neuroscience research, development of therapies for nervous system disorders, and related ethical and societal issues. She recently served as the director of the consensus study report *Preventing Cognitive Decline and Dementia: A Way Forward* and as the senior program officer for the consensus study report *Medications for Opioid Use Disorder Save Lives*. Dr. Stroud first joined the National Academies in 2009 as a science and technology policy graduate fellow. She has also been an associate at AmericaSpeaks, a nonprofit organization that engages citizens in decision making on important public policy issues. Dr. Stroud received her Ph.D. from the University of Maryland, College Park, with research focused on the cognitive neuroscience of language. She received her bachelor's degree from Queen's University in Canada.

Autumn S. Downey, Ph.D., is a senior program officer with the Board on Health Sciences Policy. She joined the National Academies of Sciences, Engineering, and Medicine in 2012 and is currently directing a consensus study on respiratory protection as well as a standing committee on the health risks of air pollution exposure for U.S. Department of State employees and their families stationed overseas. Other National Academies studies she has worked on include *Evidence-Based Practice for Public Health Emergency Preparedness and Response*; *Return of Individual-Specific Research Results Generated in Research Laboratories*; *Preventing Cognitive Decline and Dementia*; *A National Trauma Care System*; *Healthy, Resilient, and Sustainable Communities After Disasters*; *BioWatch PCR Assays*; and *Advancing Workforce Health at the Department of Homeland Security*. Dr. Downey received her Ph.D. in molecular microbiology and immunology from the Johns Hopkins Bloomberg School of Public Health, where she also completed a postdoctoral fellowship at the school's National Center for the Study of Preparedness and Catastrophic Event Response. Prior to joining the National Academies, she was a National Research Council postdoctoral fellow at the National Institute of Standards and Technology, where she worked on environmental sampling for biothreat agents and the indoor microbiome.

Sheena M. Posey Norris, M.S., is a program officer with the Board on Health Sciences Policy in the National Academies of Sciences, Engineering, and Medicine's Health and Medicine Division. Her primary interest is in policy issues related to translational and behavioral neuroscience research, neuropsychology, and global mental health. She currently works with the Forum on Neuroscience and Nervous System Disorders, previously serving as an associate program officer and a research associate, and worked on the consensus study report *Care Interventions for Individuals Living with Dementia and Their Caregivers*. Ms. Posey Norris has led and assisted in the planning of activities for the Neuroscience Forum, *Preventing Dementia and Cognitive Impairment* study, Ethical Review and Oversight Issues in Research Involving Standard of Care Interventions workshop, Forum on Medical and Public Health Preparedness for Disasters and Emergencies, *Guidance for Standards of Care During Disaster Situations* study, and Strategies for Cost-Effective and Flexible Biodetection Systems That Ensure Timely and Accurate Information for Public Health Officials workshop. Prior to joining the National Academies, Ms. Posey Norris was a research associate in the Graduate School of Nursing at the Uniformed Services University of the Health Sciences in Bethesda, Maryland. Working alongside advanced practice nurse researchers, she conducted research focusing on health-promoting behaviors of military spouses. Ms. Posey Norris received her M.S. from Saint Joseph's University in Philadelphia, Pennsylvania, in experimental psychology with an emphasis in neuropsychology. Her thesis-driven research during her graduate studies focused on the neurocognitive and balance effects of multiple concussions in young adults. Ms. Posey Norris graduated magna cum laude from Lynchburg College in Virginia with a bachelor of science in psychology and Spanish (high honors).

Andrew March, M.P.H., is a research associate for the Health and Medicine Division's Board on Health Sciences Policy (HSP), having joined the National Academies of Sciences, Engineering, and Medicine in 2018. His previous work at the National Academies includes two consensus studies on the safety and effectiveness of compounded drug preparations. Prior to coming to HSP, he performed research on sickness absence in working women at the Center for Research in Occupational Health, and he worked in the epidemiology department at the Hospital de la Santa Creu i Sant Pau in Barcelona. Mr. March obtained a B.S. in biology and Spanish from Roanoke College and an M.P.H. at the Universitat Pompeu Fabra in Barcelona.

Andrew M. Pope, Ph.D., is the senior director of the Board on Health Sciences Policy. He has a Ph.D. in physiology and biochemistry from the University of Maryland and has been a member of the National Academies of Sciences, Engineering, and Medicine since 1982, and of the Health and Medicine Division staff since 1989. His primary interests are science policy, biomedical ethics, and environmental and occupational influences on human health. During his tenure at the National Academies, Dr. Pope has directed numerous studies on topics that range from injury control, disability prevention, biologic markers to the protection of human subjects of research, National Institutes of Health priority-setting processes, organ procurement and transplantation policy, and the role of science and technology in countering terrorism. Since 1998, Dr. Pope has served as the director of the Board on Health Sciences Policy, which oversees and guides a program of activities that is intended to encourage and sustain the continuous vigor of the basic biomedical and clinical research enterprises needed to ensure and improve the health and resilience of the public. Ongoing activities include Forums on Neuroscience, Genomics, Drug Discovery and Development, and Medical and Public Health Preparedness for Catastrophic Events. Dr. Pope is the recipient of the Health and Medicine Division's Cecil Award and the National Academy of Sciences President's Special Achievement Award.

Sharyl Nass, Ph.D., serves as the senior director of the Board on Health Care Services and the director of the National Cancer Policy Forum at the National Academies of Sciences, Engineering, and Medicine. The National Academies provide independent, objective analysis and advice to the nation to solve complex problems and inform public policy decisions related to science, technology, and medicine. To enable the best possible care for all patients, the board undertakes scholarly analysis of the organization, financing, effectiveness, workforce, and delivery of health care, with emphasis on quality, cost, and accessibility. The National Cancer Policy Forum examines policy issues pertaining to the entire continuum of cancer research and care. For more than two decades, Dr. Nass has worked on a broad range of health and science policy topics that include the quality and safety of health care and clinical trials, developing technologies for precision medicine, and strategies for large-scale biomedical science. She has a Ph.D. in cell biology from Georgetown University and undertook postdoctoral training at the Johns Hopkins University School of Medicine, as well as a research fellowship at the Max Planck Institute in Germany. She also holds a B.S. and an M.S. from the University of Wisconsin–Madison. She has been the recipient of the Cecil Medal for Excellence in Health Policy Research, a Distinguished Service Award from the National Academies, the Mentor Award from the Health and Medicine Division, and the Institute of Medicine Staff Team Achievement Award (as team leader).